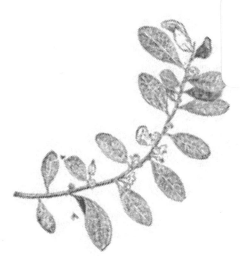

# Coca

# Divine Plant of the Incas

## W. Golden Mortimer, M.D.

Abridged
by Beverly A. Potter, PhD.

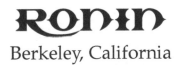

Berkeley, California

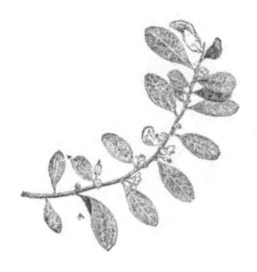

# Coca

# Divine Plant of the Incas

## W. Golden Mortimer, M.D.

Abridged
by Beverly A. Potter, PhD

# Coca
# Divine Plant of the Incas

Copyright 2017 by Ronin Publishing, Inc
ISBN: 978-1-57951-246-0

Published by
**Ronin Publishing, Inc.**
PO Box 3436
Oakland, CA 94609
www.roninpub.com

Abridged from
*History of Coca: The Divine Plant of the Incas*, by W. Golden Mortimer, M.D., And/Or Press, 1974

Production:
    Abridgement: Beverly A. Potter.
    Cover Design: Beverly A. Potter

Library of Congress Card Number:  2017958086
Manufactured in the United States by Lightning Source.
Distributed to the book trade by PGW/Ingram

# Table of Contents

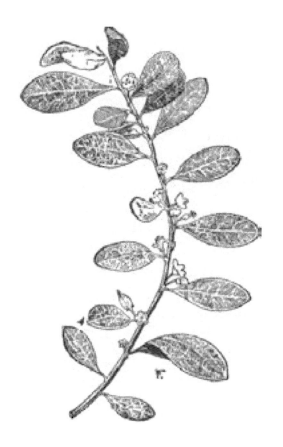

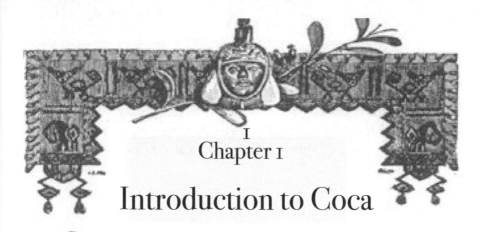

# Introduction to Coca

☞ MAN were asked what one boon he would prefer of all Earth's bounties or Heaven's blessings, his response must be—the power of endurance. The capability to patiently and persistently do best that which the laws of life or the vagaries of association necessitates. Search for this one quality has been the impetus to inspire poet and philosopher since man's first appreciation of his mortal frailty. It is something that shall check, within himself at least, the progress of time, the ravages of age, and the natural vacillation of conditions or environment. Wealth, and power, and greatness, and skill, must alike fall into insignificance without this one essential attribute to success.

The artist in impressionistic work, the poet in soulful muse, the musician in celestial chords, the soldier in the mad rush of battle, the artisan in the cleverness of device, the merchant in the intricacies of commercial problems — even the most prosaic delver in life's plodding journey— each hopes to display a virility from which the slightest weakness is deprecated as humiliating. Work, indeed, is necessary to existence.

It is the price—as the ancients considered—which the gods set on anything worth having. It is the power to do this work—to gain happiness for ourselves, which is the demand of modern necessity. To be enabled to keep active until the human machine may wear out as did the "wonderful one-hoss-shay," rather than rusting into a state of uselessness.

# Endurance

Human endurance, bounded by natural limitations, is still more closely environed by the results of a higher civilization, which presents the remarkable anomaly of two opposite conditions. While increasing, through the refinements of hygienic resources, the average term of life, it crowds man in the struggle for existence, into a condition where he is rendered less capable physically for fighting the battles into which he is thrust. So, from a natural life of pronounced perfection where his trials have been essentially muscular, he is gradually evolving into an artificial existence of eminently nervous impulse.

If this be so, then the interest in any means which shall tend to establish and maintain a balance of force, should not be merely casual, but must be earnest and persistent to any who have regard for life's best qualities, and this interest must constantly increase with the requirements of time.

Even though others may point the way, everyone must fight their own battles. To each of us the world will appear as we may shape it for ourselves—a thought poetically expressed by the composer Wagner, who said: "The world exists only in our heart and conception." This shaping, if done by weakly hands or influenced by troubled brain, may not always prove symmetrical. A sensitive imagination, sharply attune, jars discordantly amidst inharmonious surroundings, which will be all the more harshly apparent if made possible through a known impotence.

There is a fund of force communicated by the Creator to all things. It is the primal factor not only of man's existence, but of his continued being, and the activity which it generates is necessary to life, just as a cessation of energy means death. This fact has ever been so much a portion of the human mind that it requires no philosophic training to implant. It is not alone the savage who regards examples of vigor and prowess as ennobled emblems of a supreme being, while the sick or even the weak are looked upon as possessed of some evil spirit to be exorcised by priest or medicine man.

This belief, whether superstitious or not, is pre-eminent and widespread. It is not only manifested by the ignorant, but often by the educated as well. The effort to ward off disease through wearing some particular substance as a talisman is a practice prompted by this feeling, which is not wholly relegated to bygone days, and the belief in amulets, rings, or the influence of certain precious stones is still prevalent everywhere.

There is supposedly some deeply hidden

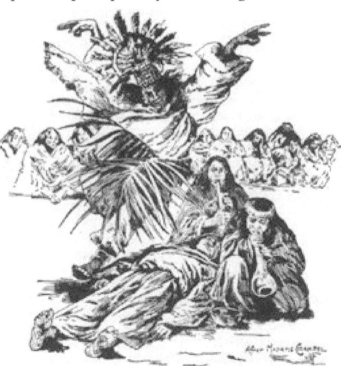

*Medicine man*

mystery about Nature in her varied presentations, which if it does not control presumably influences the curative art. It is not only those who consider that "yarbs should be gathered at a certain time of the moon," but the laity quite generally suppose there is a specific for every disease if not every condition, which if not immediately forthcoming upon inquiry must be revealed by more diligent search.

Nor is this belief—even though vague—indulged in merely by the unthinking, but everywhere about us there is a tendency against accepting rigid facts, and inevitable truths, particularly when applied to one's self. "All men think all men mortal but themselves" is surely a well founded adage. The result is a groping after that all necessary something, which shall supply this very apparent want, a craving for endurance in all we are called upon to bear.

# Elixir Vitae

There has been a numerous order of philosophers not content with simple well being, who sought for that perpetual youth—that *elixir vitae*—which might give at least prolonged existence even if not rejuvenation.

When Juan Ponce de Leon sought the *Fontaine de Jouvence* in the Island of Bimini, he failed to locate the fountain, but he did discover a land of perpetual youth. The discovery of the "Western Continent—whether due to the forethought or ignorance of Columbus, or to the hardihood of the Norsemen several centuries before his time—brought a multitude of bounties to humanity. Among these none is greater than the countless plants which have been gradually unfolded to usefulness by the processes of science.

*The properties of coca more nearly approach that ideal source of endurance than is known to exist in any other one substance.*

Particularly is this true of the economic and medicinal coca plant of South America, which on the eastern declivity of the Andes and towards the valley of the Amazon,

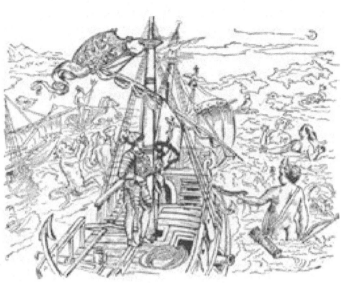

*The Discovery*

spring forth in all the luxuriance of the tropical jungle, over a vast portion of which it is supposed the foot of man has never trodden. In this locality—and among this wild profusion, grows a beautiful shrub, the leaves of which in shape somewhat resemble those of the orange tree, but in color are of a very much paler green, having that exquisite translucence of the most delicate fern.

The properties of coca more nearly approach that ideal source of endurance than is known to exist in any other one substance. Its leaves have been used by the natives of the surrounding country from the earliest recollection, as a masticatory, as a medicine, and as a force sustaining food. Its use is not confined to emergency, nor to luxury, but as an essential factor to the daily life work of these people. As a potent necessity it has been tenderly cared for and carefully cultivated through the struggles, trials and vituperation it has been the occasion of during so many hundreds of years, until to-day its cultivation forms the chief industry of a large portion of the natives and a prominent source of revenue to the governments controlling the localities where it is grown.

During the early age, when this nature's garden was unknown to the rest of the world, the Incas, who were then the dominant people of this portion of the continent, re-

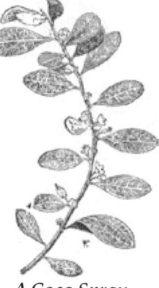

garded this shrub as "the divine plant," so all important and complete in itself, that it was termed simply *khoka,* meaning the tree, beyond which all other designation was unnecessary.

This plant, which has been described under a variety of names but now known as Coca, has appealed alike to the archaeologist, the botanist, the historian, and traveller as well as to the physician. Its history is united with the antiquity of centuries, while its traditions link it with a sacredness of the past, the beginning of which is lost

*A Coca Spray*

in the remoteness of time. So intimately entwined is the story of Coca with these early associations—with religious rites, with superstitious reverence, with false assertions and modern doubts—that to unravel it is like to the disentanglement of a tropical vine in the primitive jungles of its native home.

# Source of Knowledge

Antedating historical record Coca was linked with the political doings of that most remarkable people of early American civilization who constituted the Incan dynasty. Since the conquest of Peru it has continued to form a nec-

essary factor to the daily life work of
the Andean Indians, the descendants
of this once noble race. So important
has it been held in the history of its
native land that it has very fittingly
been embodied in the escutcheon of
Peru, along with the vicuna and the
horn of plenty, thus typifying endurance with the versatile riches which
this country affords.

*Unlike the Mexicans, these people had no picture writings to tell their doings in a series of hieroglyphics, nor had they a written language.*

The first knowledge to the outer
world concerning Coca followed
Pizarro's invasion of Peru, though the actual accounts of
its properties were not published until some years after
the cruel murder of Atahualpa—commonly regarded as
the last Incan monarch. The effort made by the Spanish to
implant their religion raised the cross and shrine wherever possible, which necessitated the founding of numerous
missions, in charge of fathers of the church.

These men in holy orders were often as tyrannical as
those who bore arms, yet fortunately there were some in
both classes less cruel, men of liberal attainments who appreciated the importance of preserving the traditions and
records of this new country. To the writings of some of these
more kindly disposed personages, as well as to the earnest
labors of a few young nobles who were in the army of invasion, whose spirit for a conservative exploration was greater
than for destructive conquest, we are indebted for the facts
which form the foundation of this early history.

Many of these writers had personally seen the result of
the Incan civilization before its decay, and had opportunity
to collect the native stories, as retold from father to son,
through generation after generation, oral tradition being
the early Peruvian method for continuing a knowledge of
events. Unlike the Mexicans, these people had no picture
writings to tell their doings in a series of hieroglyphics,

*The Spanish idea of conquest was to establish a complete mastery over the Peruvians; the Indians were regarded as slaves to be bought, sold, and used as such.*

nor had they a written language. But the story of this once mighty empire is told in its wonderful ruins, and through the relics of skillfully moulded pottery, and textile fabrics in exquisite designs, which all indicate a remarkable civilization. Historical facts were related by regularly appointed orators of phenomenal memory, who on all state occasions w⁷ould recount the occurrences of the preceding reign, being aided in this recital by a novel fringelike record of colored cords, known as the *quipu.*

By the aid of this, as a sort of artificial memory, they told, as a monk might tell his beads. The various knots and several colors of the contrivance designating certain objects or events. In all these relations the Coca leaf was repeatedly and reverently alluded to as a most important element of their customs, as well as of their numerous feasts and religious rites.

The Spanish idea of conquest was to establish a complete mastery over the Peruvians; the Indians were regarded as slaves to be bought, sold, and used as such. In view of these facts it is not difficult to understand that as Coca was constantly employed among the natives, its use was early questioned and condemned as a possible luxury, for it was not considered a matter worthy of inquiry as to any real benefit in a substance employed by slaves.

So superficial were the observations made by some of the early writers that the fact of this neglect is most apparent. Thus, Cieza de Leon, a voluminous writer on Incan customs, mentions as a peculiar habit of the natives: "they always carry a small leaf of some sort in the mouth." Even so experienced an observer as Humboldt, in his writings of many years later, did not recognize the true quality of Coca, but confounds the sustaining properties of the leaf as due to the alkaline ashes—the *Llipta*—which is chewed with it. He refers to the use of this lime as though it belonged to the custom of the clay eaters of other regions, and suggests that any support to be derived from it must necessarily be purely imaginary.

# Chewing Condemned

It is not surprising that Coca chewing, if superficially viewed, would be condemned. The Spanish considered it merely an idle and offensive habit that must be prohibited, and at one time it was even seriously suggested that the plants should be uprooted and destroyed. But it was soon seen that the Indians could not work without Coca, and when forced to do so were unequal to the severe tasks imposed on them. As, however, the local tribute to the authorities demanded from all able bodied laborers a fixed amount of work, it was soon appreciated as a matter of policy that the use of Coca must at least be tolerated in order that this work should be done.

Then the Church, which was from the invasion an all-powerful force in this new country, exacting and relentless in its demands, saw an imaginative evil in this promiscuous Coca chewing. If Coca sustained the Indians, it was of course a food, and its use should not be allowed before the holy eucharist. Necessity brought forth a deliverer from this formidable opponent, and it was represented that Coca was not an aliment, and so its use was reluctantly permitted.

But now came still another effort to prohibit it, from moral motives. The Indian believed in Coca, he knew that it sustained him without other food in his arduous work, but it had been conclusively shown that it was not a food, and so could not sustain, hence his belief was false, superstitious, even a delusion of the devil to warp the poor

Indian from the way he should go. Greed, however, pre-
dominated, as gold has ever been a convincing factor, and
as the Indian could do most work when supplied with
Coca, its use was finally allowed unrestricted, and to-day
a portion of Coca is given to all Andean laborers as part of
their necessary supplies.

## Spirit of Antagonism

So it will be seen that like all scientific advances which
have been made, since Prometheus incurred the wrath of
Jove by stealing fire from the gods to put life in mortals,
until the present time, Coca has not been admitted to ac-
ceptance unassailed. That spirit of antagonism that seems
rampant at the very suggestion of progress has caused
its allies to rehabilitate and magnify the early errors and
superstitions whenever opportunity might admit, together
with those newer accessions of false premises engendered
through shallowness of investigation. Every department
of science has been subjected to similar instances of annoyance, though it would appear that medicine is particularly
more subject to such influence. At first a partisan sentimen-
tality, with an exaggeration which provokes condemnation
and often results in oblivion, or what in calmer judgment
may be a true balance of worth.

It is amusing to now look back at some attacks which
were hurled against substances that all the world today
considers as necessities. The anaesthetic use of chloroform
was at first regarded as unholy because it was asserted
man is born unto pain as he is unto sin, and so should
bear his necessary sufferings in a holy and uncomplaining
manner.

Every physician frequently meets with just such original and plausible opposition to suggested remedies to-
day. When in 1638 Cinchona was introduced into Europe

under the name of "Jesuits' powder," it was vigorously denounced as quackery. So great was the prejudice that sprang up against it, even among those eminent physicians whom we now look back upon as the fathers of medicine, that when Chiftelius, in 1653, wrote a book against "the bark," he was complimented as though he had relieved the world of a monster or a pestilence. For years it was not countenanced by "the faculty," and the various arguments then advanced concerning its supposed action form curious reading. The opposition to vaccination, in 1770, was something that excited not only the protests of physicians and learned societies, but the clergy and laity as well. The College of Physicians shook its wise head and refused to recognize Jenner's discovery. The country doctor was considered something of a bore. Innumerable other instances might be cited to testify to this negative spirit prompted by any advance.

Among food products, the humble potato when introduced into Scotland, in 1728, was violently denounced as unholy because "not mentioned in the Bible." It was asserted that it was forbidden fruit, and as that was the cause of man's first fall, to countenance its use would be irreligious. In France, so strong was the feeling against the introduction of potatoes that Louis XVI and his Court wore the flower of the plant as a *boutonniere* to give the much opposed—but desirable—potato at least the prestige of fashion.

Tea, coffee and chocolate have each been denounced, and from very high sources too. "A lover of his country," as he designated himself, in 1673, proposed to Parliament "the prohibition of brandy, rum, coffee, chocolate and tea, and the suppressing of coffee houses. These hinder greatly the consumption of barley, malt and wheat, the product of our land." Here would seem to be an ulterior motive that is almost suggestive of the commercial spirit often now displayed, which would suppress one product that another may be permitted to flourish regardless of merit.

As an argument against the pernicious and growing tendency to use tea and coffee, after they had been rendered palatable through knowing how to use them, a Dr. Duncan, of the Faculty of Montpelier, in 1706, wrote: "Coffee and tea were at the first used only as medicine while they continued unpleasant, but since they were "made delicious with sugar, they are become poison."

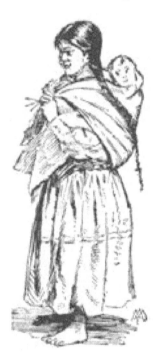

The *Spectator* of April 29th, 1712, urges against the dangers of chocolate as follows: "I shall also advise my fair readers to be in a particular manner careful how they meddle with romances, chocolates, novels, and the like inflamers which I look upon as very dangerous to be made use of during this great carnival." Opinion on these beverages is not unanimous today even, as harmless as they are commonly considered. Alcohol and tobacco of course have come in for an unusual share of denunciation, and the argument is not yet ended. From these through the entire range of stimulant-narcotics, each has excited such vigorous protests that the very term stimulant is considered by some as opprobrious. How real must be the merit that can withstand such storms of abuse, and spring up, perennially blooming, through such opposition!

*An Andean Nurse*

Coca is unparalleled in the history of plants, and although it has been compared to about every plant that has any stimulating quality, it is wholly unlike any other. In this comparison tobacco, kola, tea, mate, guarana, coffee, cacao, hashish, opium, and even alcohol, has been referred to. It has been made to bear the burden of whatever evils lurk in any or all of these, and has unjustly been falsely condemned through such association.

That Coca is chewed by the South American Indians and tobacco is smoked by the North American Indians, that Coca is used in Peru and opium or betel is used in the East—is a fair example of this comparison. It no more nearly resembles" kola—with which it is often carelessly confounded, the properties of which are chiefly due to caffeine—than through the allied harmony of its first syllable. While a similarity to various substances taken as beverages is possibly suggested through the fact that Coca is sometimes drunk in decoction by the Peruvians.

## Cerebral Effects

The cerebral effects of Coca are entirely different from hashish or opium, and its stimulant action in no way comparable to alcohol. I do not mention these substances to decry them, but merely to illustrate the careless comparisons which have been advanced, through which imperfect conclusions must necessarily be drawn. Then again, there is an unfortunate similarity between the pronunciation of the names Coca, and cocoa or cacao—the chocolate nut, and coco—the coconut, which has occasioned a confusion of thought not wholly limited to some of the laity.

The fact remains that though Coca is used by millions of people, it is not generally known away from its native country. Even many physicians constantly confound it with allied plants of dissimilar properties or with substances of like sounding name. That this is not simply a broad and hasty statement may be illustrated by the

*The cerebral effects of Coca are entirely different from hashish or opium, and its stimulant action in no way comparable to alcohol.*

following fact. The writing of this work was prompted by the immense divergence of published accounts regarding the efficacy of Coca, in view of which an effort was made to learn the result of its use among a representative class of practitioners, each of whom it was presumed would be well qualified to express an opinion worthy of consideration.

An autograph letter, together with an appropriate blank for reply, fully explaining the desirability for this data, was prepared, of which ten thousand were sent out. These were addressed to professors in the several medical colleges, and to those prominent in local medical societies—all eminent in practice. Many did not reply, while of the answers received, fully one half had—"never used Coca in any form." Of the balance, many are—"prejudiced against its use," through some preconceived notion as to its inertness, or through some vague fear of insidious danger which they were not prepared to explain, and even preferred not to inquire into, being—"satisfied it is a dangerous drug."

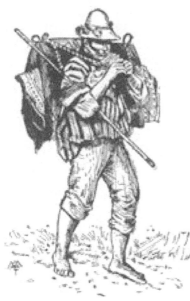

*A Coca Carrier*

There are others who inadvertently confound Coca with some of the confusional drugs already referred to or with cocoa. That this was not merely an apparent fault, through some slip of the pen in hasty writing, is shown by direct answer to the question as to the form of Coca found most serviceable, stating so and so's "breakfast *coca*" is used in place of tea or coffee. In some instances the benefits of Coca were enlarged upon with an earnestness that was inclined to inspire confidence. The physiological action was gone into minutely and its therapeutic application extolled, only to conclude with the amazing statement that the fluid extract, the wine, or "breakfast *coca*" were interchangeably used, thus displaying a confusion worse confounded which might be amusing if not so appalling.

# Confusion

These confusional assertions display one source of error, yet in view of the entwined facts concerning Coca through literature and science it must emphasize the unfortunate neglect of observation, and the refusal to recognize advancement manifest even in this progressive age—among some whose duties and responsibilities should have spurred to a refinement of discernment. It is suggestive of the anecdote told by Park, who when in his Eastern travels asked some Arabs what became of the sun at night, and whether it always was the same sun, or was renewed each day, was staggered with they reply: "such a question is foolish, being entirely beyond the reach of human investigation."

Replies fully as surprising were received in this inquiry. Several have taken the "moral" side of the question quite to heart, and expressed a belief that through advocating the popularizing of Coca, I was tending to contribute to the increase of a pernicious and debasing habit which was already undermining the morals of the community. Others again have tried to show me the error I had fallen into when speaking of the dietetic uses of Coca. As one gentleman emphatically expressed it: "This is some terrible mistake, you are confounding Coca with Cocoa! Cocoa is used for food, but Coca—*never.*" So that even that part of my investigation pursued among modern medical men has not been as easily carried out as might at first be supposed. There has been the same or similar ignorance and error to sift apart from truth as encompassed the early historical associations of the plant.

This unfortunate confusion is probably to be accounted for because Coca was largely used empirically and without a proper appreciation of its physiological action before its properties were fully known. Writers who have described its local use among the Andean Indians have advanced statements regarding its sustaining qualities which have not been verified by some observers elsewhere located, even though these latter may have carried out a careful line of physiological experimentation. The explanation of this has only recently been determined, but is now known to be due to the extreme volatility of the associate principles of Coca.

Recent, or well-cured and properly preserved Coca is wholly different from leaves which have become inert through improper treatment. Then again as our botanical knowledge of this plant has increased, it has indicated that not all leaves termed Coca are such. The family to which the classic leaves of the Incans belong has many species. Among the particular species of Coca there has only quite recently been determined several varieties.

The properties of these differ materially according to the presence or absence of certain alkaloidal constituents. Some of the early experiments upon the properties of Coca were made at a time when these facts were unknown, and with this, was the added disadvantage of the impossibility of then obtaining appropriately preserved Coca in the open markets. Not only may the substance examined have been inert, but through different observers using different varieties of Coca the conclusions could not possibly agree.

Unfortunately because of the apparent carefulness of research these early statements were accepted and given a wide publicity, and so from the marvelous apparent benefits of Coca among native users to the absolute inertness pronounced by some foreign observers, there has been a very wide space for the admission of much distrust. The busy physician must commonly accept the result of the

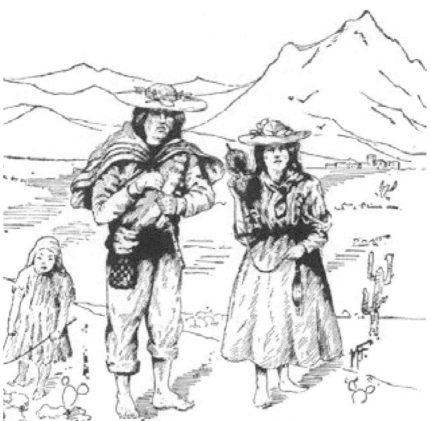

*Descendants of the Incans*

provings of the experimentalist, and amidst so much doubt it may have seemed easier to set aside a possible remedy than to have personally verified the assertions. Indeed, trial has only too often depreciated hopes from a happy realization of the wonderful properties attributed to the use of native Coca on the Andes, to a realization of the uncertainty of the marketed product at command. In which connection it may not seem too astonishing to say I know of an instance where senna leaves were sold by a wholesale drug house for "fresh Coca leaves," while I doubt if any drug house would make a distinction in offering the casual purchaser any variety of Coca at hand.

It was because of "this uncertainty"—of the conflicting stories and the impossibility to unify facts—that interest in Coca, which had been stimulated in Europe by Dr. Mantegazza about 1859, soon declined until disuse almost left it in forgetfulness. About this time Niemann, then a pupil of Professor Woehler, isolated the alkaloid cocaine from the leaves, and attention was again awakened to the possible usefulness of the parent plant.

# Cocaine

It was supposed, however, that the active principle to which all the sustaining energy of Coca was due had been discovered in cocaine. Here again was a radical error, and an unfortunate one as it has since proved, to still more confound an intricate problem. This is particularly serious because it is widely accepted as truth, not only among many physicians, but also because it has been spread by this misunderstanding through the secular press, and so falsely impressed the laity.

As a result, cocaine has been promiscuously used as a restorative and sustainer under the supposition that it is but Coca in a more convenient and active form. The evils that have followed this use have fallen upon Coca, which has often been erroneously condemned as the cause. It is owing to the wide spread of this belief as well as its resultant evil and because of the difficulty for the lay mind to appreciate the radical difference between Coca and cocaine—between any parent plant and but one of its alkaloids—that it must necessarily require long and persistent effort on the part of educated physicians to explain away this wrong, to reassure those who have been falsely informed as to the real merits of Coca, and so reflect credit upon themselves through the advocacy and use of a really marvelous remedy.

The truth cannot be too forcibly impressed, that co-caine is but one constituent, and no more fully represents Coca than would prussic acid—because found in a minute quantity in the seeds of the peach—represent that luscious fruit. In emphasizing this a recent investigator who passed a long period in the Coca region, studying as a scientist the peculiarities of the plant, and watching as a physician its effect upon native users of the drug, says: "With certain restrictions it may be said that the properties of cocaine, re-markable as they are, lie in an altogether different direction from those of Coca as it has been reported to us from South America."

So it will be seen that because of misconstruing early tales and superstitious beliefs, because inert leaves have not yielded results of the sound plant, because some dif-ferent variety has not yielded the same results as the clas-sic type, because one of its alkaloids does not represent the whole, the parent plant is condemned. Because of this ignorance of certain investigators the historical accounts of the use of Coca and its sustaining qualities among the natives, have been set down to exaggeration or absolute fabrication. As one physician replying to my inquiries would have others believe: "The Indians are great liars." Thus from ignorance, neglect or from false conception, Coca was either wholly ignored or little understood in a popular way, until in 1884 a renewed interest was awak-ened through the discovery of the qualities of cocaine as an anaesthetic in the surgery of the eye. Then, as though forgetful of all preceding investigation or condemnation, a renewed discussion commenced regarding the asserted qualities of Coca, the failure to realize them, and the prob-able source of potency of the plant as represented by co-caine.

This was followed by frequently reported accounts of a new and terrible vice which was springing up every-where—the so-called "cocaine habit." For this Coca was

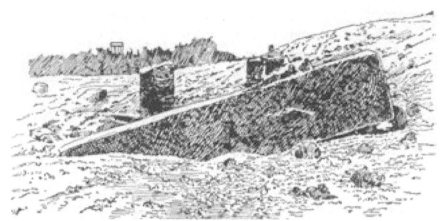

*Mammoth stone at Baalbek, Syria. Similar to manßy monoliths in this land of the Incas.*

condemned as its enemies pretended to now see the real element of perniciousness. Yet before cocaine was ever dreamed of and during the long centuries in the history of Coca, not one case of poisoning from its use has ever been recorded. The accusation of "habit" had, however, long before been erroneously directed against the leaves. But of this, one who wrote scientifically and extensively on Peru after personal observation, sets forth his conclusions in the following positive way:

*"Coca is not merely innocuous, but even very conducive to health." He even calculated the improbability of harm by estimating, if an Indian reached the age of one hundred and thirty years—which seems to be the only "habit" to which these people are addicted beside the "habit" for hard work—he would have consumed two thousand seven hundred pounds of leaves, an amount sufficient to have quite fully determined all pernicious possibilities. Indeed, to think of Coca as an injurious substance suggests the character in one of Madison Morton's farces who wished to "shuffle off" speedily, and determined to chew poppy heads "because poppy heads contain poppy seeds, and poppy seeds eaten constantly for several years will produce instant death."*

The theory has been advanced that because cocaine is one of the chief alkaloids of Coca, it represents whatever sustaining quality the leaf can possibly have, and-manufacturers base their choice of leaves upon the percentage of cocaine determined by assay. But this is not in unanimity with the selection of the native users of Coca, any more than would the quality of a choice tobacco leaf be governed by the amount of nicotine it contains.

The fact is the Andean Indian selects Coca that is rich in the more volatile associate alkaloids and low in cocaine. It is what is known as the sweet in contradistinction to the bitter-leaf, which latter is made bitter by the large amount of cocaine it contains. On this very point an authority says:

*"It only remains for me to point out that the relative amount of cocaine contained in native Coca leaves exerts no influence in determining the Indian's selection of his supply. As a matter of fact, the ordinary conditions to which the leaves are subject during the first two or three months after they are gathered have but little effect upon their original percentage of cocaine. The Indian, however, makes his selections from among such leaves with the greatest care, eagerly seeking the properly dried leaves from some favorite cocal, whose produce is always most readily brought out, and absolutely rejecting other leaves, notwithstanding that the percentages of cocaine may be almost identical."*

# Sensational Assertions

The absolute reliance of the Andean Indians upon Coca not only for sustenance, but as a general panacea for all ills, has naturally led them to feel a superstitious regard for the plant. This reverence has descended to them from the Incan period, during which the shrub was looked upon as "a living manifestation of divinity, and the places of its growth a sanctuary where all mortals should bend the knee." However much the Incas reverenced Coca they did not worship it: it was considered the greatest of all natural productions, and as such was offered in their sacrifices. Their ceremonial offerings were made to thair conception of deity—the sun, which they held to be the giver of all earthly blessings.

The ideas of moral depravity, and the fears of debasing habit following the use of Coca, have sprung from false premises and early misconceptions as to the true nature of the plant. As a matter of fact, neither "habit," as that is understood, nor poisoning has ever been recorded against Coca among the natives where it has been continued in use for centuries. Those early writers on Andean customs who allude to Coca chewing all speak positively against any evil result following its use. One physician, after being intimately associated among the natives for nearly a year, where he had witnessed the constant use of Coca, failed to find a single case of chronic cocaism, although this one subject chiefly occupied his attention, and he searched assiduously for information. Speaking of the amount used, he says: "what it does for the Indian at fifteen it does for him at sixty, and a greatly increasing dose is not resorted to. There is no reaction, nor have I seen any of the evil effects depicted by some writers and generally recorded in books."*cocaism*" means the habit of chewing coca leaves.

# The Spanish Object

The early objections by the Spanish against the use of Coca were rather as persecutions, intended to still further oppress this conquered race by taking from them what was looked upon as an idle and expensive luxury. But Coca-chewing could never be an expensive luxury in a country where it grows wild, and where it is given by those in charge of laborers as a regular portion of each man's daily supplies. The later cries against its perniciousness, as has been shown, were based wholly upon the action of cocaine following the widespread use of that alkaloid as a local anaesthetic.

Reports in the medical press of injurious effects from the use of cocaine all date from the period when the entire medical world was active in the discussion of the merits of this great boon to minor surgery. It would seem that many then rushed into print without regard to method so long as something was said about the all-absorbing topic of the time, which might direct a portion of attention to themselves. A new opportunity had arisen when old tales and early prejudices might be again reiterated concerning Coca. The lay press was not slow to take up the sensational side of the subject, and the "cocaine habit" soon became a well-determined condition in theory, and a fashionable complaint.

I have personally investigated a number of such reported cases and

*The ideas of moral depravity, and the fears of debasing habit following the use of Coca, have sprung from false premises and early misconceptions as to the true nature of the plant.*

in every instance have found either that it was a condition engrafted upon some previous "habit" in a nervous subject, or else that the report was absolutely false. There is no motive—as the lawyers would say——for the offense, there is no reason for the establishment of a habit such as exists in the case of alcohol or opium. The fact is there exists a certain class of subjects who are so weak in will power, that if they should repeat any one thing for a few consecutive times they would become habituated to that practice.

But such cases are the exceptions, and have no especial bearing upon Coca. In the collective investigation among several thousand physicians, this matter was particularly impressed as an important point of inquiry and the answers sustained the facts already explained, that a Coca habit has never existed. During the early part of 1898 a case was reported very sensationally in the secular press regarding a Dr. Holmes who had died in an asylum at Arden-dale, N. Y., a hopeless wreck as a result of cocaine habit. I communicated with the physician in charge of that institution and was promptly assured "Dr. Holmes did not die as a result of 'cocaine habit,' nor had he ever been addicted to it."

## Attacks Survived

That Coca has survived the attacks which have been periodically hurled against it during several hundred years, and that its use is not only continued, but its therapeutic application constantly increasing, must suggest to the thinking mind that it is possessed of remarkable value. It has continued with the Andeans not because they have formed a "habit" for it, not because it fills their minds with that ecstatic and dreamful bliss as habit drugs would do, but because experience has taught them that they can perform their work better by its use.

There is a practical utility in it that will be seen when detailing some of the customs of these people, is so exact that they measure their distances by the amount of Coca that they chew instead of by the rod and chain, or chronometer. Their use of this plant is continued day after day during a long lifetime, yet the amount of Coca that sustains them in young adult life is not increased in their old age. Its force product is a constant factor, just as a given amount of water under proper *That any plant or substance that has been continued in daily use by millions of people over a vast territory, for many hundreds of years, should have so long remained unrecognized by the world at large seems almost incredible.* conditions will make a known amount of steam. The fuel taken and the work performed is always the same, other conditions being equal.

Can it be presumed for a moment that if this general and persistent use of Coca is a depraved habit, sapping the best of moral qualities, even manhood, unfitting its users to perform their duties, that these people would be capable of the immense amount of physical work which they do? It is known to be a fact by those employing large forces of workmen in the Peruvian mines, that the Indian would not and could not perform the tasks he is set to under the exposure he is subjected to without Coca. This is well shown by contrast when foreigners are compelled to work with them, and are unable to perform an equal amount of labor to theirs until they too have recourse to the use of Coca. Thus it must be seen that Coca is as worthy today as it was in the time of the Incas of being termed the "divine plant." It is Nature's best gift to man. It neither morally corrupts nor undermines manhood, or vitality, as is well shown in these Indians, who are long-lived and are held by those who know them best, to be conservative, respectful, virtuous, honest and trustworthy, addicted to hard work—and the use of Coca, that they may more thoroughly and successfully do that work.

That any plant or substance that has been continued in daily use by millions of people over a vast territory, for many hundreds of years, should have so long remained unrecognized by the world at large seems almost incredible. Yet the fact is undoubted, as has been shown, and Coca is even today unknown to a great majority of not only the masses, but of physicians. Since the date of the Conquest, the constant use of Coca leaves by the Indians has been frequently referred to by travellers, often superficially, yet commonly agreeing as to its sustaining qualities. But so wonderful have these accounts seemed that their simple relation has usually excited doubt rather than belief. They have been looked upon as "travellers' tales," relations due to an imagination, which possibly had been expanded by the conjoined influence of a rarefied atmosphere, and an exalted desire to enhance the wonders of travel. So from doubting qualities which were long looked upon as improbable or unexplainable, and from the inaccuracies recorded by those who affected scientific research on old leaves, it was but a simple step to relegate the very existence of the plant to the legendary.

It has been shown in outline how varied were the causes to account for this unbelief, and the consequent neglect which followed. Primarily to superficial observation on the part of early explorers in an unknown country, where consideration for mere existence was to the unacclimated often of the first importance. Added to this was the conservative reticence of the Indians, and their superstitious regard for this plant so intimately linked with their religious and political life. This alone was sufficient to prevent the ready acquirement by travellers of a detailed knowledge of the use of Coca, or even of native customs and the reason for them.

Here was sufficient possibility for hasty conclusions, aside from the forceful attacks of both Church and State against what they were pleased to regard as the continuance of a superstitious practice or vulgar habit, which possibly linked the desires of these people whom they hoped to Christianize, with an idolatrous past. Then, too, there existed as now, a class of zealots seeing imaginative wrong in every custom, who would have every act discontinued simply because it is done, in dread of some direful consequence which may result. In furthering each of these negative influences, theories were often advanced at variance with existent facts, and so many conflicting tales and much confusion has resulted.

Absurd stories have been published, and these again copied without apparent attempt at verification, the whole establishing a falsity from which there has grown a diversity of opinion wholly inconsistent with the exact requirements of science. Meanwhile the rapid progress of the world in exploration often engrossed attention to the exclusion of details. The demand of commercial interests, for broad facts and immediate results in the amassing of wealth, diverted attention from the tales of travellers or the disputes of scientists. But as a higher civilization demands the resources of the universe to maintain its conditions, the secret of Nature's gift to the Andean could not remain long hidden, and the means which afforded support for these simple people was recognized as of possible benefit to the rest of the plodding, toiling world.

As Coca was shown to be a necessity to the Andean in his toilsome travels of exposure, its adaptability was suggested to other members of the human family elsewhere located who are comparatively as subject to privation and hardship as are these primitive people. Even in our great cities among modern resources the labor is exacting and exhaustive, and whether the work done be a strain of muscular exertion or a prolonged mental effort, the resultant

wear and tear is similar, and the conditions are to be met
by recourse to the most expedient means available.

Unfortunately the Spanish invasion of Peru so largely destroyed all native records that it has been difficult
to readily retrace a continued history of the remarkable
people of this early civilization, among whom our story
of Coca must begin. But from the period of the Conquest,
after it had been made known to the outer world Coca was
frequently sung in poetry or recounted in the tales of travellers. It however continued, since the privilege was extended from its early users to their descendants, to almost
exclusively be enjoyed by these people until less than half
a century ago.

In properly determining the benefits of Coca it seems
desirable to trace back its historical connections and its
associations between past uses and present necessities,
as well as to inquire into those surroundings that have
prompted its use and called for its continuance. This must
necessarily lead us through many interesting fields where
the view may seem remote from our narrative, yet is essential to the full understanding of a story the first impulse for
which was generated in the horrors of the Conquest.

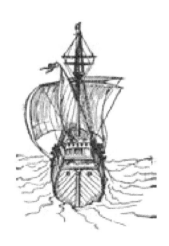

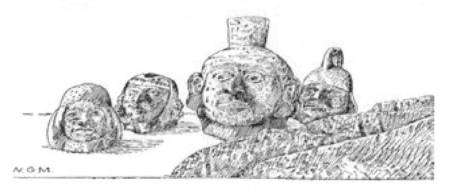

## Chapter 2

# History

**D**ARWIN gave prominence to the doctrine of Malthus that organic life tends to increase beyond means of subsistence, and emphasized a statement of Spencer that in the struggle for existence only the fittest survive. Among economic plants we have no more pronounced example of these laws than is illustrated in the Coca plant. It has stood not only the mere test of time, but has survived bitter persecutions wherein it was falsely set up as an emblem of superstition, in a cruel war of destruction when the people among whom it was held as sacred were exterminated as a race.

Coca has marked the downfall of one of the most profound examples of socialism ever recorded in history, and has outlived the forceful attacks of Church and State which were maliciously hurled against it as an example of idolatry and perniciousness. These attacks were the outgrowth of a shallowness of thought, intermingled with the prevalent prejudices of the several important epochs of its history. In the earliest literature concerning Peru we trace the beginning of this element of superstition toward Coca, for it was presumed there could be no good custom followed by the Indians. The entire aboriginal American race was regarded by the invaders as little more than savage devils worthy only of extermination. Thus Pedro Cieza de Leon, who wrote at the time of the Conquest, garnished his tales with pictures and stories of the Prince of Evil, with whom the Indian was inferred to be in close compact.

Cieza was a mere boy of fourteen when he embarked with Don Pedro de Heredia, in 1532, to seek fortune in the New World. When we consider that the conceptions of this writer were only such as might be inspired by the rough and rugged opportunities which camp life offered, it certainly seems remarkable that he had the foresight to compile so acceptable a journal of the early Peruvians. The seriousness with which he undertook this task, and his exactitude in recording current events, may be appreciated from his statement: "I noted with much care and diligence, in order that I might be able to write with that truth which is due from me and without any mixture of inaccuracies."

Heredia founded the city of Cartagena, in the province of Tierra Firma, as Panama was originally termed, and after Cieza had spent five years of life there, he enlisted under Pedro Vadillo in a desperate exploit across the mountains of Ahibe and through the valley of Cauca and Popayan. Subsequently we find this boy historian marching with Robbdo and then serving under Belalcazar, until, as the chronicler states, "he, too, became entombed in the bellies of the Indians"—for they were marching through a country of savages who were cannibals.

Cieza was first intimately associated with Peruvian affairs in the campaign with Gasca, at the final rout of Gonzalo, and he afterward travelled under this first President of the Royal Audience through the interior of Peru. Having compiled an extensive notebook of the country and the doings of the times, which was to form a connecting link between the Incas and the Spanish invaders, he returned to Lima by way of the coast from Arequipa, from whence

he sailed for Spain September
8, 1550. The events during
seventeen years of travel he
has recounted in his chronicles
with remarkable minuteness.

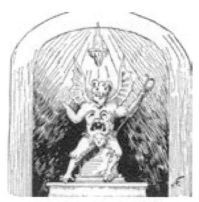

There was a prejudice and
superstitious credulity among
the Spanish conquerors for
all the customs of the Incas.
The bigotry of the time is well
illustrated in a story told of
Columbus. On the return from

*Early Spanish Devil*

his first voyage he took with him to Spain several Indians,
who were baptized at Barcelona, where one of them shortly
afterward died, and lierrera, referring to this nearly three
hundred years after, tells us this Indian "was the first native of the New World who ever went to Heaven," though
no intimation is made as to the probable destination of the
millions of Americans who had preceded him.

Amidst such prejudices, it is not surprising that the
Coca plant so prized by the Indians was deemed by the
Spanish unworthy of serious consideration, and that it was
looked upon by them merely as a savage means of intoxi-
cation, or at best a mere source of idle indulgence among a
race they so much despised.

Throughout his writings Cieza refers frequently to
Coca, though he has not given any very concise botanical
description of the plant, referring more particularly to its
common use. In the first part of his chronicles of Peru, he
says: "In all parts of the Indies through which I travelled
I noticed the Indians delighted to carry herbs or roots in
their mouths; in one province of one kind, in another another sort, etc. In the Districts of Quimbaya and Anzerma
they cut small twigs from a young green tree, which they
rub against their teeth without cessation.

*The Incas regarded Coca as a symbol of divinity, and originally its use was confined exclusively to the royal family.* In most of the villages subject to the cities of Cali and Popayan they go about with small Coca leaves in their mouth, to which they apply a mixture which they carry in a calabash, made from a certain earth-like lime. Throughout Peru the Indians carry this Coca in their mouths; from morning until they lie down to sleep they never take it out. When I asked some of these Indians why they carried these leaves in their mouths, which they do not eat, but merely hold between their teeth, they replied that it prevents them from feeling hungry, and gives them great vigor and strength. I believe that it has some such effect, although perhaps it is a custom only suitable for people like these Indians. They so use Coca in the forests of the Andes, from Guamanga to the town of La Plata.

# The Leaf Called Coca

The trees are small, and they cultivate them with great care, that they may yield the leaf called Coca. They put the leaves in the sun, and afterwards pack them in little narrow bags containing a little more than an arroba each. This Coca was so highly valued in the years 1548, '49, '50 and '51 that there was not a root nor anything gathered from a tree, except spice, which was in such estimation. In those years they valued the repartimientos of Cuzco, La Paz and Plata at eighty thousand dollars, more or less, all arising from this Coca. Coca was taken to the mines of Potosi for sale, and the planting of the trees and picking of the leaves was carried on to such an extent that Coca is not now worth so much, but it will never cease to be valuable. There are some persons in Spain who are rich from the produce of this Coca, having traded with it, sold and resold it in the Indian markets."

# Valued Gift

The sovereign could show no higher mark of esteem than to bestow a gift of this precious leaf upon those whom he wished to endow with an especial mark of his imperial favor. So when neighboring tribes who had been conquered by the Incas, acknowledged their subjection and allegiance, their chiefs were welcomed with the rank of nobles to this new alliance and accorded such honors and hospitalities as gifts of rich stuffs, women and bales of Coca might impress.

At the time of Mayta Ccapac—the fourth Inca, his queen was designated Mama Coca — "the mother of Coca," as the most sacred title which could be bestowed upon her. From so exalted a consideration of the plant by royal favor, it was but a natural sequence that the mass of the people should regard Coca as an object for adoration worthy to be deemed "divine." Cristoval Molina, a priest at the hospital for the natives at Cuzco, from whose work[5] we have drawn our account of the rites and festivals of the Incas, has related the method of using Coca by the high priests in conducting sacrifices. Just as Cieza, with the material instinct of the soldier, saw only the physical or superstitious element in the use of Coca among the Indians, so this priest traced for us its spiritual association with the ceremonies of the people. Thus there was early interwoven the factors of an adoration of the masses, and a blending of these with a religious regard for Coca, for the teachings of the Church were engrafted upon existing customs in order to hold the people.

The first scientific knowledge of Coca published in Europe was embodied in the writings of Mcolas Monardes, a physician of Seville, in 1565, from material possibly gained from Cieza, though it would seem that he had intimately examined the Coca shrub. A translation of this work was made a few years later by Charles l'Ecluse—a botanist and director of the Emperor's Garden at Vienna—which was published in Latin at Antwerp, and this is often quoted as the earliest botanical reference to Coca. The Kew Library possesses a translation of this book, "made into English" by John Eramp-ton and printed in black letter with the curious title: *"Joyful Neivs out of the Newe Founde Worlde, wherein is declared the Virtues of Hearbes, Treez, Oyales, Plantes and Stones."*

As showing the discernment in this botanical description of Coca made so many years ago, it may not be uninteresting to read a paragraph translated from the very language of Monardes:

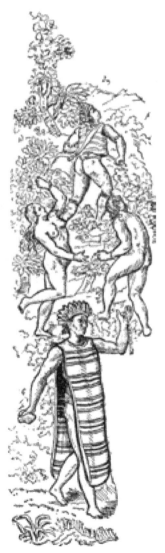

*"This plant Coca has been celebrated for many years among the Indians, and they sow and cultivate it with much care and industry, because they all apply it daily to their use and pleasure. It is indeed of the height of two outstretched arms, its leaves somewhat like myrtle, but larger and more succulent and green (and they have, as it were, drawn in the middle of them another leaf of similar shape); its fruit collected together in a cluster, which, like myrtle fruit, becomes red when ripening and of the same size, and when quite ripe it is black in color. When the time of the harvest of the leaves arrives, they are collected in baskets with other things to make them dry, that they may be better preserved, and may be carried to other places."*

This description will hold equally good to-day. The peculiar leaf within a leaf arrangement formed by the curved lines running on either side of the midrib, being a marked characteristic of Coca.

When Hernando Pizarro returned to the court of his king, with the first fruits of the golden harvest from the New World, he probably took with him specimens of Coca. This plant could not have failed to have awakened at least the curiosity of the invaders, because of the numerous golden duplications of the Coca shrub and of its leaf that had been found in the garderis of the Temples of the Sun, at Cuzco and elsewhere among the royal domains of the Incas. So that whatever the prejudices may have been regarding the use to which Coca was put by the Indians, these golden images at least would prove sufficient to excite admiration and comment.

Another voluminous writer upon the early Peruvians is Joseph de Acosta, a Jesuit missionary who made a passage across the Atlantic in 1570, which he assures us:—"would have been more rapid if the mariners had made more sail." After his arrival at Lima he crossed the Andes by the lofty pass of Pariacaca to join the Viceroy Toledo, with whom he visited every province. In the higher altitudes of the mountains the party suffered severely from the effects of the rarefied atmosphere, with which he was afterwards prostrated upon three successive occasions, while he also was severely annoyed from snow blindness, for which he relates a homely remedy offered him by an Indian woman, who gave him a piece of the flesh of the vicuna, saying, "Father, lay this to thine eyes, and thou shalt be cured." He says: "It was newly killed and bloody, yet I used the medicine, and presently the pain ceased, and soon after went quite away."

Father Acosta was a man of great learning, an intelligent observer, and had exceptional opportunities for collecting his information. His work on the Natural History of the Indies ranks among the higher authorities. He has

given a very extensive description of Coca, and, referring
to its employment, says: "They bring it commonly from
the valleys of the Andes, where there is an extreme heat
and where it rains continually the most part of the year,
wherein the Indians endure much labor and pain to enter-
tain it, and often many die. For that they go from the Sierra
and colde places to till and gather them in the valleys; and
therefore there has been great question and diversity of
opinion among learned men whether it were more expedient to pull up these trees or let them grow, but in the end
they remained.

## Much Esteemed

The Indians esteemed it much, and in the time of the Incas
it was not lawful for any of the common people to use this
Coca without license from the Governor.  They say it gives
them great courage, and is very pleasing unto them. Many
grave men hold this as a superstition and a mere imagination. For my part, and to speak the truth, I persuade not
myself that it is an imagination, but contrawise I think it
works and gives force and courage to the Indians, for we
see the effects which cannot be attributed to imagination,
so as to go some days without meat, but only a handful of
Coca, and other like effects. The sauce wherewith they do
eat this Coca is proper enough, whereof I have tasted, and
it is like the taste of leather. The Indians mingle it with the
ashes of bones, burnt and beat into powder, or with lime,
as others affirme, which seemeth to them pleasing and of
good taste, and they say it doeth them much good. They
willingly imploy their money therein and use it as money;
yet all these things were not inconvenient, were not the
hazard of the trafficke thereof, wherein so many men are
occupied. The Lords Yncas used Coca as a delicate and royal thing, which they offered most in their sacrifice, burning
it in honor of their idols."

Again, when speaking of the importance of the trade in Coca, he says: "It seems almost fabulous, but in truth the trafficke of Coca in Potosi doth yearly amount to above half a million of dollars; for that they use four score and ten or four score and fifteen thousand baskets every year."

## Potosi Mines

This extensive mining centre in the southern part of Bolivia is some three hundred miles south of Sandia, which is today the very heart of the Coca region of Caravaya. These mines were at an altitude of seventeen thousand feet, and Garcilasso says the Indians applied the term Potosi, literally a hill, to all hills.   In the Aymara tongue Potosi means, "he who makes a noise," and the Indians have a legend which suggests the derivation of the name from such a source. When Huayna Ccapac caused his people to search this mountain for silver, a great noise came from the hills warning the Indians away, as the protecting genius destined these riches for other masters. Within a short time after the Incas had discovered silver here over seven thousand Indians were at work mining the precious ore.

The Spaniards were not slow to recognize this vast store of treasure, and in their haste to accumulate the wealth which they had come so far to secure they forced the Indians to labor in veritable slavery through an enactment which drafted a certain number from each of the adjoining provinces. This law, known as the *mitta,* instituted under Toledo, required all Indians between the ages of eighteen and fifty to contribute a certain labor, which amounted to eighteen months during the thirty-two years in which they were liable. For this they were paid twenty reals a

*Within a short time after the Incas had discovered silver here over seven thousand Indians were at work mining the precious ore.*

week, and a half real additional for every league distant from the village of Potosi. During the year 1573 the draft of Indians for this labor amounted to 11,199, while a hundred years later—in 1673—it drew only 1,074, showing that cruelty and hardship had depopulated the province nearly ninety per cent.

So extensive were the mining operations at Potosi that the place had the appearance of a great city. Every Saturday the silver was melted down and the royal fifth was set aside for the Spanish crown, and although this amounted

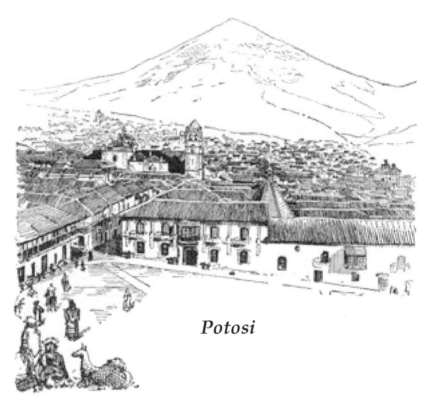

*Potosi*

during the years 1548 to 1551 to three million ducats, it was considered the mines were not well worked. In those times the markets or fairs were important functions, and that of Potosi was looked upon as the greatest in the world. It was held in the plains near the town, and there the transactions in one day were said to amount to from twenty-five to thirty thousand golden pesos, Coca being a prominent commodity in the reckoning, owing to its absolute necessity in the arduous work exacted from the Indians.

Because of this need the highest price was obtained for Coca in this region, where every indication was presented for its use—the extreme altitude of the mines, the mental dejection of slavery, and the enforced muscular task of the Indian with insufficient food. This labor was found to be utterly impossible without the use of Coca, so that the Indians were supplied with the leaves by their masters, just as so much fuel might be fed to an engine in order to produce a given amount of work. Garcilasso tells us that in 1548 the workers in these mines consumed 100,000 *cestas* of Coca, which were valued at 500,000 piasters.

This absolute necessity was the sole reason for the Spanish tolerance to the continuance of Coca; they saw that it was indirectly to them a source of wealth, through enabling the Indians to do more work in the mines. As the demands of labor increased the call for Coca, situations for new cocals, where a supply of the plant could be raised to meet this want, were pushed further to the east of the Andes, in the region of the montana.    To make favorable clearings numerous tribes of savage Indians, who had not been previously subdued by the Incas, were driven from the Peruvian tributaries of the Amazon further into the forests.

Agustin de Zarate, who was *contador real*, or royal comptroller, under the first Viceroy, Blasco Nunez Vela, in his history of the discoveries of Peru, in writing of Coca, says: "In certain

*This labor was found to be utterly impossible without the use of Coca, so that the Indians were supplied with the leaves by their masters, just as so much fuel might be fed to an engine in order to produce a given amount of work.*

valleys, among the mountains, the heat is marvellous, and there groweth a certain herb called Coca, which the Indians do esteem more than gold or silver; the leaves thereof are like unto Zamake (sumach); the virtue of this herb, found by experience, is that any man having these leaves in his mouth hath never hunger nor thirst."

Garcilasso Inca de la Vega—as he delighted in terming himself—has very rightly been classed as an eminent authority on Incan subjects. His father, who was of proud Spanish ancestry, illustrious both in arms and literature, came to Peru shortly after the Conquest, served under Pizarro, and after the overthrow of the empire, when the Incan maidens were assigned to various Spanish officers, his choice fell upon the niece of Inca Huayna Ccapac, who in some manner had been preserved from the massacre which had followed upon the death of her cousin, Atahualpa. It seems fitting that a son of such parentage should embody in his writings facts which he had obtained from both branches of the family tree, and because of this his work is accepted as a reliable presentation.

That this Incan author was well qualified to speak upon Coca there can be no doubt, for he owned an extensive cocal on the River Tunu, one of the tributaries of the Beni— which drains the montana for Paucartambo—where there are still numerous cocals. This plantation was started in the twelfth century during the reign of Inca Rocca, when that king sent his son with fifteen thousand warriors to conquer the savage tribes of Anti-suyu.

Lloque Yupanqui advanced to the River Paucartambo and thence to Pillcu-pata, where four villages were founded, and from Pillcu-pata he marched to Havisca, and here in the year 1197 was located the first Coca plantation of the montana on the eastern base of the Andes.[10] This Incan plantation became an inheritance of Garcilasso from his father, but was forfeited by the historian because of his parent's early defection to the cause of Gonzalo.

The work of Garcilasso is interesting as embracing with the relation of others that of Father Bias Valera, whose manuscripts have since been lost, and in this embodied record we have the only available account of one who was a close observer of Incan customs during a residence of many years in Peru. To the peculiar wording of the work of this author we may trace an oft-repeated error regarding the Coca shrub, which he describes as "a bush of the height and thickness of the vine." Whether this designation of vine refers to the grape, which in some vineyards is grown as a low clump resembling a bush, or whether the term vine simply alludes to the delicate nature of the Coca shrub, can only be inferred. It has introduced a source of inaccuracy among some who have since drawn their description of the plant from this record. One author has even amplified this early comparison by saying that the Coca bush twines about other plants for support.

Valera, in describing the leaves of Coca, says: "They are known by Indians and Spaniards alike as *Cuca,* delicate, though not soft, of the width of the thumb and as long as half a thumb's length, and of a pleasant smell." In his day the Indians were so fond of Coca that they preferred it to gold, silver and precious stones. He has given us a careful account of the diligence which is necessary in the several stages of its cultivation and the importance of the final gathering of the leaves, which he says, "they pick one by one by hand and dry them in the sun." He, however, wrongly viewed the method of use, and supposed that the leaves were merely chewed for their flavor and that the juice was not swallowed.

Referring to the general employment of Coca for a variety of purposes, he says:

*"Cuca preserves the body from many infirmities, and our doctors use it pounded for applications to sores and broken bones, to remove cold from the body or to prevent it from en-*

*tering, as well as to cure sores that are full of maggots. It is so*
*beneficial and has such singular virtue in the cure of outward*
*sores, it will surely have even more virtue and efficacy in the*
*entrails of those who eat it I" Nor did this observant author fail*
*to recognize another important use in which this famous plant*
*was practically serviceable. A tax of one-tenth of the Coca crop*
*was set apart for the clergy, of which he says: "The greater part*
*of the revenue of the bishops and canons of the cathedrals of*
*Cuzco is derived from the tithes of the Coca leaves."*

There is a marked contrast between the open, conscientious
manner of Valera's writings with that of other Spanish
authors, who displayed an abhorrence for all the customs
of the Indians. Thus Cieza, reflecting this superstitious
prejudice, tells us that the old men of every tribe actually
conversed with the arch-enemy of mankjnd. Referring to
the Incan rite of burying bags of Coca with their dead, as
a symbol of support for the departed in a journey to the
eternal home, he mockingly says, "as if hell was so very
far off." The good *padre*, in his appeal for the continuance
of Coca, has shown a liberality for such a period of bigotry
which might be well for the consideration of others in even
this more enlightened age. Thus he writes:

*"They have said and written manythings against the little*
*plant, with no other reason than that the Gentiles in ancient*
*times, and now some wizards and diviners, offer Cuca to the*
*idols, on which ground these people say that its use ought to*
*be entirely prohibited. Certainly this would be good counsel*
*if the Indians offered up this and nothing else to the devil,*
*but seeing that the ancient idolaters and modern wizards also*
*sacrifice maize, vegetables and fruits, whether growing above*
*or under ground, as well as their beverage, cold water, wool,*
*clothes, sheep and many other things, and as they cannot*
*all be prohibited, neither should the Cuca. They ought to be*
*taught to abhor superstitions and to serve truly one God,*
*using all these things after a Christian fashion."*

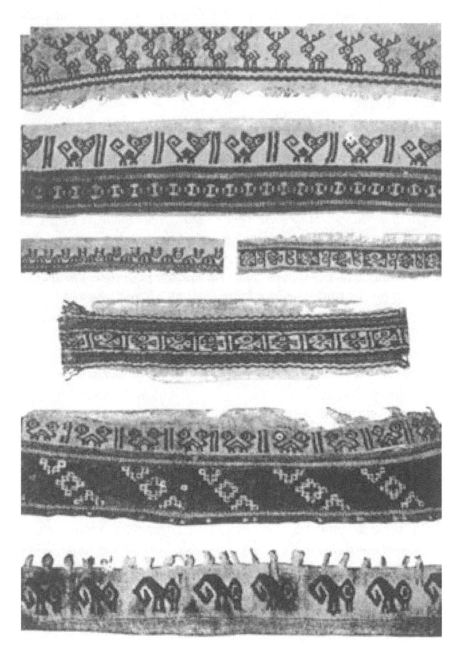

*Borders of Incan Tapestry*

Garcilasso has added to this account some further par-
ticulars made familiar to him through his intimate acquain-
tance with the cultivation and care of Coca. In his quaint
verbiage, which has possibly suffered through translation,
he says of the shrubs:

*"They are about the height of a man, and in planting them
they put the seeds into nurseries, in the same way as in
garden stuffs, but drilling a hole as for vines. They layer the
plants as with a vine. They take the greatest care that no
roots, not even the smallest, be doubled, for this is sufficient
to make the plant dry up. When they gather the leaves they
take each branch within the fingers of the hand, and pick
the leaves until they come to the final sprout, which they do
not touch, lest it shoidd cause the branch to wither. The leaf,
both on the upper and under side, in shape and greenness,
is neither more nor less than that of the arbutus, except that
three or four leaves of the Cuca, being very delicate, would
make one of arbutus in thickness. I rejoice to be able to find
things in Spain which are appropriate for comparison with
those of that country—that both here and there people may
know one by another. After the leaves are gathered they put
them in the sun to dry. For they lose their green color, which
is much prized, and break up into powder, being so very delicate, if they are exposed to damp, in the cestas or baskets in
which they are carried from one place to another. The baskets
are made of split canes, of which there are many of all sizes
in these provinces of the Antis. They cover the outside of the
baskets with the leaves of the large cane, which are more than
a tercia wide and about half a vara long, in order to preserve
the Cuca from wet, for the leaves are much injured by damp.
The basket is then enveloped by an outer net made of a certain fibre."*

Keferring to the extreme care essential for its preservation,
this Incan author concludes: "In considering the number of
things that are required for the production of *Cuca*, it would
be more profitable to return thanks to God for providing all

things in the places where they are necessary than to write concerning them, for the account must seem incredible."

Father Thomas Ortiz, who accompanied Alonzo Niiio and Luis Guerra in their expedition in 1499, described the use of Coca by the natives along the coast of Venezuela under the term *hayo*.™

Antonio de Herrera, who was royal historian under Philip II, drew his facts from correspondence with the *con-quistados*, and his history, which is divided into eight decades, covers the period of the Spanish discoveries. In speaking of the customs of the northern provinces, he refers to "the herb which on the coast of the sea is called *hayo*."[10] The word *hayo* has been shown to belong to the vocabulary of the Chib-chas and is generally applied to Coca by several tribes bordering upon the northern coast of South America.

Among some of the earlier Spanish writings of this section Coca is alluded to as "hay," and doubt has been expressed as to whether this is identical with *hayo*, presumably derived from *agu*, to chew; but the absence of the final vowel, according to a writer who is familiar with this region, does not signify, while it is absolutely certain that all the species of *Erythroxylon* which are today used in Venezuela and along the Caribbean Sea are termed *hayo*. Even the *Erytliroxylon cumanense*, HBK, is called by this name and not that of *ceveso*, as mentioned in the description published by Kunth.

The account which Ortiz gives of the plant used by the Indians of Chiribiche does not exactly correspond with the Coca shrub, though what he says of the leaves and their use among the Indians is correct. Gomara, in speaking of the customs of the *Cumana*, confirms the account given by Ortiz. At present Coca is not very extensively grown through Venezuela. The ancient cocals on the peninsula of Guajira are becoming extinct on account of excessive drought, while the cultivation of tobacco has proved a more profitable industry and is better adapted to the climate.

We know that prior to the Conquest, the province of the Incas extended north to Quito, having been conquered by Huayna Ccapac some years before for his father, Tupac Inca Yupanqui, by which conquest the powerful State of Quito, which rivaled Peru in wealth and civilization, was united to the Incan Empire. When Huayna Ccapac succeeded his father, this newly acquired kingdom became his seat of government, and here with his favorite concubine, the mother of Atahualpa, he spent the last days of his life.

Because of this removal of imperial influence far from the original home of the empire at Cuzco may be attributed one source of the final weakness of the Incas, for it may be recalled that at the time of Huayna Ccapac's death the kingdom, which now extended over such immense territory, was for the first time divided under two riders, one-half being given to his son, Huasca, and the other half to his son Atahualpa. It therefore seems quite probable that as the interests of the government extended northward the customs of the people of the lower Andes should follow, and be propagated among a people where similar conditions called for whatever beneficial influence might be derived from the use of Coca. From Quito travel northward, aided by the canoe navigation of the Cauca and Magdalena rivers, would rapidly carry the customs of the people of the south to the northern coast, where, as shown by early historical facts, commerce was so extensive as to favor the adoption of the habits of the interior.

There are still many tribes along the Sierra Nevada of Santa Marta who have preserved their ancient customs and habits from prehistoric times, for it is known that the Spanish were never able to completely attain possession of this region. It has been suggested that these Indians had never been subject to a king as were the Incas, while their country was so extremely fertile that when pursued by the Spanish they merely destroyed their homes and took up habitations elsewhere, depending upon a bountiful tropical vegetation for their support.

# Subjection

In marked contrast to the Indians of New Grenada, the Peruvians were accustomed to subjection under their Lord Inca, and at the time of the Conquest they were obliged to submit themselves to their new masters, for if they abandoned their homes and the lands which they had cultivated to flee to the barren mountains or snowy plains they must also give up their means for subsistence. Piedrahita speaks of the use of Coca along the northern coast, and says that the leaves were chewed by the Indians without lime, an addition which he suggests was carried from the Incan domains to the northern Indians by the Spaniards after the Conquest.

The expedition of the French mathematician, La Conda-mine, which went to Quito in 1735 to measure an arc of the meridian in the neighborhood of the equator, and thus verify the shape of the earth, was made memorable through a host of important scientific discoveries, primary among which was the introduction of many new plants into Europe; among these was caoutchouc or india rubber. Accompanying this expedition was Antonio d'Ulloa, a Spanish naval officer; Godin, Bouguer and the botanist, Joseph de Jus-sieu, whose name is associated with the classification of Coca. Condamine was the first man of science who examined and described the *quinquina* tree of Loxa, of which Linnajus in 1742 established the genus *Cinchona*.

Jussieu travelled on foot as far as the forests of Santa Cruz de la Sierra, collecting botanical specimens from the

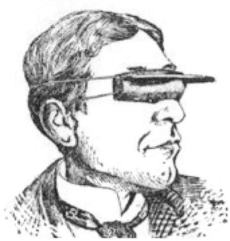

*Esquimo Sun Shield*

richness of the Peruvian flora. Many of his exploratory trips were hazardous in the extreme, and in 1749, while crossing the Andes to reach the Coca region of the Yungas of Coroico, he nearly lost his life. Added to the dangers of the route the glistening brilliancy of the sun reflected from the snow seemed to threaten him with blindness. In the Arctic region travellers are subject to a similar discomfort, and commonly wear a visor-like protector to shield their eyes. The sun shade illustrated is carved from wood with slots cut beneath the peak to permit of vision.

Jussieu sent specimens of the Coca shrub to Paris, and these, examined and described by the explorer's brother An-toine, were afterward preserved in the herbarium of the Museum of Natural History there, and have served as classic examples of many subsequent studies of the plant. But the glory of meritorious labor pursued through great trial and privation was not to be enjoyed by this explorer. Just as many another collector before and since his time has suffered the loss of treasures when work was about completed, so this intrepid botanist lost the choice gatherings of fifteen years through robbery, under the belief that his boxes contained a more merchantable wealth than plants. In 1771, after an absence of thirty-four years, Jussieu was taken home, bereft of reason, as a result not alone of hardships, but from that unfulfilled desire which makes the soul sick, and he died in France, leaving many manuscripts, which are still unpublished.

The Jussieus were a family of botanists for several generations; contemporary with them were several noted naturalists who followed their classification. Among these, Augustin Pyrame Candolle, of the College of France, and Antonio Jose Cavanilles, a Spanish ecclesiastic, each described Coca from the examples which had been sent by Joseph.

Many interesting accounts have been written of the expedition of La Condamine, and as a result of these early researches several of the powers have been prompted to send botanical expeditions to the South American forests. Among these there is given in the writings of Captain Don Antonio d'Ulloa a brief account of the country of Popayan, in the jurisdiction of Timana. While following Father Valera's description of Coca, he adds: "It grows on a weak stem, which for support twists itself around another stronger vegetable like a vine. The use the Indians make of it is for chewing, mixing it with chalk or whitish earth called *mambi*.™

They put into their mouths a few Coca leaves and a suitable portion of *mambi,* and chewing these togetlier, at first spit out the saliva which that mastication causes, but afterwards swallow it, and thus move it from one side of the mouth to the other till its substance be quite derived, then it is thrown away, but immediately replaced by fresh leaves."

He confounds Coca with betel, saying: "It is exactly the same as the betel of the East Indies. The plant, the leaf, the manner of using it, its qualities, are all the same, and the eastern nations are no less fond of this betel than the Indians of Peru and Popayan are of their Coca; but in other parts of the province of Quito, as it is not produced, so neither is it vised." But he was conscious of the physiological effects of Coca from its employment, and wrote: "This herb is so nutritious and invigorating that the Indians labor whole days without anything else, and on the want of it they find a decay in their strength. They also add that it preserves the teeth sound and fortifies the stomach."

The early writings upon Coca were not, however, all of foreign authorship. Peru numbered among her men of letters a noted physician and statesman who drew his facts from a keen observation of the people of whom he wrote. I refer to Dr. Don Ilipolito Unanue, of Tacna, whose name is intimately linked with the political and educational history of Peru. He published the *Mercurio Peruana*, the first number of which appeared in January, 1791, a paper which gave an impetus to the writings of his countrymen, in which there are many interesting details of Peruvian customs.

From his political interests in a land where insurrection was a common occurrence, Dr. Unanue could appreciate the advantage possible from the use of Coca in the army. He tells an incident of the siege of La Paz, in 1771, when the inhabitants, after a blockade of several months, during a severe winter, ran short of provisions and were compelled to depend wholly upon Coca, of which happily there was a stock in the city. This apparently scanty sustenance was sufficient to banish hunger and to support fatigue, while enabling the soldiers to bear the intense cold. During the same war a body of patriot infantry, obliged to travel one of the coldest plateaus of Bolivia, found itself deprived of provisions while advancing in forced marches to regain the division. On their arrival only those soldiers were in condition to fight who had from childhood been accustomed to always carry with them a pouch of Coca.

# Prejudice Difficult To Eradicate

That early prejudice is difficult to eradicate, is shown in the writings of some who, having given the facts of the use of Coca, then seem to apologetically qualify their reference to its support as a mere delusion. Thus Dr. Barham, writing of Coca in 1795, says:

*"This herb is famous in the history of Peru, the Indians fancying it adds much to their strength. Others affirm that they use it for charms. Fishermen also put some of this herb to their hook when they can take no fish, and they are said to have better success therefor. In short, they apply it to so many uses, most of them bad, that the Spaniards prohibit the use of it, for they believe it hath none of these effects, but attribute what is done to the compact the Indians have with the devil."*

But if there was prejudice on the part of the Spanish against native customs, the Indians resorted in kind with an equal antipathy against all Spanish innovations. This has been exhibited in the strong objection which the Indians have made to 'using cinchona bark. Humboldt, who forms the connecting link between the eighteenth and nineteenth centuries in our history of Coca, has referred to this, as have several other observers. It is quite probable, however, that this was a pretended prejudice openly expressed, while secretly the Indians acknowledged the benefits of the bark, which the story of its introduction relates as having been presented to the Countess of Chinchon by a descendant of the Incas.

Humboldt traveled extensively through the province of Popayan in 1801. In describing the use of Coca among the early inhabitants he asserted that several

*Augustin Pyrame De Candolle*

species of *Erythrox-ylon* were in use, chiefly *E. Ilondense*.
His conception of the benefit of Coca, however, was confined to a belief that it was the lime rather than the leaf
which formed the element of sustenance. Since his time so
many travellers directed attention to the fact that the Indians were supported by some mysterious principle, that
European investigators began to question whether this was
really due to the Coca leaf or some secret admixture. The
popular interest at the time was well set forth by an English writer, who appreciating the importance to be expected to a modern civilization from the introduction of the
method of the Andean, said:

> *"While not yet fully acquainted with the secret with which
> the Indians sustain power, it is certain they have that secret
> and put it in practice. They masticate Coca and undergo
> the greatest fatigue without any injury to health or bodily
> vigor. They want neither butcher nor baker, nor brewer, nor
> distiller, nor fuel, nor culinary utensils. Now, if Professor
> Davy will apply his thoughts to the subject here given for
> his experiments, there are thousands even in this happy land
> who will pour their blessings upon him if he will but discover
> a temporary anti-famine, or substitute for food, free from all
> inconvenience of weight, bulk and expense, and by which any
> person might be enabled, like the Peruvian Indian, to live and
> labor in health and spirits for a month now and then with-
> out eating. It would be the greatest achievement—whatever
> a London alderman might think—ever attained by human
> wisdom."*

In the early days when the traveller crossed the Andes in
the region of Popayan, he was carried in a chair on the
back of an Indian. The roads, then dangerous at all times,
became practically impassable in unsettled weather; and
the journey of twenty leagues from Popayan to La Plata
on the Magdalena Paver occupied twenty to twenty-two
days. The conditions were such as to call forth all reserve
of endurance, and not only the Indian, but. the traveller

found relief and sup-
port during severe trials
from the use of Coca.
Bonny-castle, a captain
of royal engineers, in referring to the use of Coca
by the natives in these
journeys, confounds it
with betel, following the
earlier error of Ulloa.

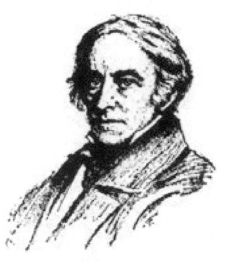

The wonderful en-
durance of the guides
and mail carriers trav-
elling through passes of          ***Karl Von Martius***
the Cordilleras where a
mule could not go, has been a frequent topic for comment
by many writers, and though so often repeated is still
wonderful. Stevenson, who was for twenty years in Peru,
during which period he held many political appointments
under the captain-general of Quito, in describing the customs of the people, refers to the runners, or *chasquis,* carrying letters from Lima, a distance of upward of a hundred
leagues, without any other provision than Coca, just as did
their predecessors centuries before in the time of the Incas.

The attention of the English people was particularly
directed to this sustenance of the Andeans by the fact that
one of their countrymen, who became a prominent partic-
ipant in the Peruvian war of independence, boldly announced his belief in the support which his troops derived
from the chewing of Coca. General Miller not only employed Coca in his army during the campaign of 1824, but
so freely acknowledged the benefit he derived from its use
that he established a warm sympathy with the natives, and
it became desirable for an Englishman travelling through
the interior to announce himself as a countryman of Miller, when he was sure to receive:—"the best house and the

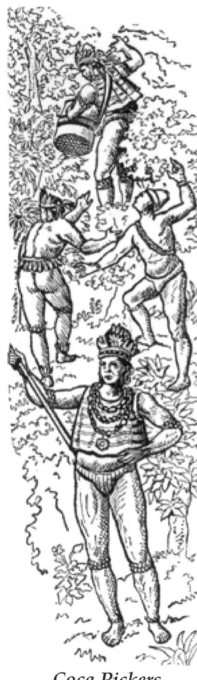

*Coca Pickers*

best fare that an Indian village could afford."

The frequent occurrence of similar allusions in the writings of South American travellers to the sustaining influence of Coca emphasized by repetition the importance of this propserty, while happily the developments of time have removed the stigma of a fabulous or superstitious element from its use.

Among the eminent scientists who wrote of Coca during the next decade were Poeppig, Tschudi, Martius and Weddell. Eduard Poeppig was a German naturalist who travelled in Peru and Chili between the years 1827 and 1832. Poeppig was not an enthusiastic admirer of Indian customs, and endeavored to associate some pernicious after effect with the sustaining power of Coca, which he considered comparable with opium. In referring to this statement Dr. Weddell—a more careful observer, held that while possibly there had been some abuse in the intemperate use of Coca by Europeans, there was in no instance the injurious results which had been asserted. He believed, as many of the Indians had assured him, that Poeppig had been led into error through generalizing exceptional occurrences

Perhaps the Swiss naturalist, Yon Tsclmdi, who visited South America in 1838, has been more frequently quoted in a popular way regarding Coca, than any other Peruvian traveller. Throughout his writings he testifies enthusiastically and forcibly for Coca, not only as employed among the natives, but from personal benefit in sustaining respiration when ascending to high altitudes. He tells of an Indian sixty-two years old who labored for him five days and nights without food and with but two hours' sleep each night, yet was still in condition to accompany him over a journey of twenty-three leagues, through which he jogged along afoot as rapidly as the mule carried his master, though depending wholly upon Coca for his sustenance. A similar experience has been reported by many travellers, for this custom is still practiced by the Indian guides.

Von Tsclmdi concluded that Coca is nutritious in the highest degree.

"Setting aside all extravagant, and visionary notions on the subject, I am clearly of the opinion that moderate use of Coca is not merely innocuous, but that it may even be very conducive to health. In support of this conclusion, I may refer to numerous examples of longevity among Indians, who, almost from the age of boyhood, have been in the habit of masticating Coca three times a day, and who in the course of their lives have consumed no less than two thousand seven hundred pounds if at the age of one hundred and thirty, and they commenced masticating at ten years — -one ounce a day, yet nevertheless enjoy perfect health."

This testimony is repeatedly added to by observers in various sections of South America. Martins, in describing Coca as used throughout western Brazil, under the name of *ypadu*, or *ipadu*, called attention to the wonderful effect which

the powder of the dried leaves has upon the nervous system, especially on the brain, and recommended the adoption of Coca among the treasures of materia medica.

Many theories have been advanced, to explain the
ability of the Indian to endure through long journeys and
hard labor, without other support than is afforded through
chewing Coca. It has been suggested that this hardihood
and abstinence is due to habit and to vigorous development. But on the contrary the Indian is muscularly weak,
and while training and habit
*With a handful of* may have much to do with
*roasted corn and only* his fortitude, he constantly
*Coca an Indian will* requires the physical support
*travel a hundred miles* afforded by Coca. Dr. Valdez,
*afoot, keeping pace* in writing of the use of Coca—
*with a horse or mule.* or *"folha sagrada,"* as he terms
it, has emphasized this: "The
Indian is naturally very voracious, and loses his strength
when abstaining from the leaves. With a handful of roasted
corn and only Coca an Indian will travel a hundred miles
afoot, keeping pace with a horse or mule."

The researches of Dr. Weddell, a French botanist who went
to South America with the scientific expedition of Count de
Castelnaii, sent out by Louis Philippe in 1845, not only confirmed, but harmonized the writings of those who had   previously described the sustenance from this leaf.

Though his researches were chiefly directed to the
study of cinchona, his travels necessarily took him through
the Coca regions, lie visited the forests of Caravaya and
Sandia, and the valley of Santa Ana, near Cuzco, all prolific Coca districts, where he had favorable opportunity for
carefully examining the method of raising and preparing
the leaf for the market. The commendations and carefully
written details of this scientist gave a marked and added
interest abroad to the economic use of Coca.

These facts of travellers and naturalists have been elaborated by the historians, and Prescott, in his story of the *Conquest of Peru*, and Helps, in the *Spanish Conquest in America*, have embodied the salient points regarding the efficacy of Coca, or *Eryihroxylum Peruvian-um*, as the former as well as Miller terms it. Mr. Prescott had voluminous manuscripts at his disposal in the compilation of his famous work, with ample opportunity to verify statements. He particularly alludes to the assertion of Poeppig as to the injurious influence of Coca, of which he says: "Strange that such baneful properties should not be the subject of more frequent comment by other writers! I do not remember to have seen them even adverted to."

A scientist who rendered particularly valuable services in the interest of cinchona was the English botanist, Richard Spruce, whose name is associated with one variety of Coca. He went to South America in 1849, and for ten years devoted himself to a study of the flora along the Amazon and tributary streams. His researches were varied and extensive, particularly in mosses and the *Ilepatica:* Among his collections were examples of twenty or more native languages, while the botanical specimens numbered thousands of species, examples of which have enriched the herbarium at Kew. Dr. Spruce remarked the dependence for support which the Indians of the Rio Xegro placed in the constant chewing of a certain variety of Coca. The powdered leaves were mixed with tapioca and the ashes of *imbauba—cecropia peltata—*as a *Uipfa*. With a chew of this in his cheek, he said, the Indian would travel two or three days without food or without a desire to sleep.

Though many expeditions had been made through Peru in behalf of other powers, it was not until 1854 that the United States government sent an exploratory expedition under Lieutenants Gibbon and Ilerndon in search of the source of the Amazon. Many facts pertaining to the diatoms of the Indians, and the use of Coca in the districts

these officials travelled, are embodied in their entertaining
narrative report to Congress. Ilerndon, while in the valley
of Chin-cliao, where the cultivation of Coca commences in
the northern montaiia—between the central and eastern
Cordilleras—mentions a visit to Senor Martins at his *hacienda* of Cucheros. The Sehor told him this *quebrada* produced seven hundred *cargas,* or mule loads of two hundred
and sixty pounds each, yearly. The value of such a crop
at Huanuco, estimated at three dollars the *arroba* of twenty-five pounds, would make the gross yield $21,840, which,
requiring seven hundred mules for transportation at a rate
of $4 apiece, would reduce the earnings to about $19,000,
though many of the small farms in the neighborhood then
sold their Coca on the spot for two dollars the *arroba.*

At Tarma the expedition separated, Herndon to follow the head waters of the Amazon, while Gibbon was to
seek the source of the Madre de Dios—or, as it is termed
in Quichua, *Amaru Mayu,* or snake river—and explore the
Bolivian tributaries. The route led Gibbon to Cuzco, where
he had opportunity to observe the industry about the royal
city among cocals which had been plantations ever since
the time of the Incas. As a rule Coca is grown in a small
way by farmers who till their own land, but in a frontier
settlement was seen a cocal which gave employment to a
hundred laborers.

There is a legend of the naming of the southern tributary of the Amazon by Padre Kevello. The savage Chun-
chos, who are much feared in this region, at one time
made a raid upon a neighboring settlement, killed the
Christianized Indians, and destroyed their little church,
throwing the sacred images into the stream. These were
carried to the *Amaru Mayu,* where they rested upon a rock
and afforded a suggestive hint for christening these waters,
"Madre de Dios," by which name they have since been
known. The most inveterate *coqueros* consider the Coca
grown on the tributaries of the Madre de Dios, in Peru, to

be superior to that produced along the waters of the Beni, in Bolivia. These two streams have their origin near to each other, between the gold washings of Tipuani and Caravaya, but a separating ridge of mountains causes the Madre de Dios to flow directly into the Amazon, while the Beni goes to the Madeira River.

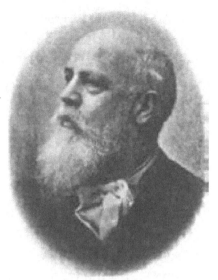

*Angelo Mariani*

The markets of La Paz are well supplied with fruits and vegetables from Yungas on the Beni, and at one time nearly five hundred thousand baskets of Coca of seventy pounds each were annually produced there.

Of the wages paid to Coca cultivators who are unfortunate enough to oe compelled to farm for others, it is related that the superintendent of a cocal below the valley of Cochabamba in Bolivia, received his shelter, scant cotton clothing, and fifteen dollars a year, a pittance sadly reduced by tithes to the Church. Yet this man was not happy! He longed for the gay days in his native town of Socaba, where he might indulge in an occasional cup of *chicha* instead of impersonating "the man with the hoe" all day long in the Coca patch.

An epoch in the introduction of Coca to the medical men of Europe was marked by the *prize essay* of Dr. Paolo Mantegazza, published at Milan on his return after a residence in Peru, where he had been engaged in practice. He refers to the employment of Coca not only as a medicine but also as an article of food, a use not confined to the rich, like luxuries usually, but which, on the contrary, is prevalent among the working Indians, who enjoy Coca as a nutriment and restorative. So that a laborer in contracting for work bargains not only for the money which he shall receive but the amount of Coca which shall be furnished him.

*"The child and the feeble old man seize with eagerness the leaves of the wonderful herb, and find in it indemnification for all suffering and misery."*

Contemporary with these writings was the labor of Mr. Clements Markham, who visited Peru in 1859, for the purpose of collecting specimens of cinchona to establish its cultivation in India. This gentleman is a scholar of South American literature, and has rendered available to English readers the knowledge of the doings of the Spanish conquerors through translations of their early writings. His intimate study of Incan customs and the affairs of modern Peru, enables authoritative statements.

Of Coca he says:

*"Its properties are to enable a greater amount of fatigue to be borne with less nourishment, and to prevent the occurrence of difficulty in respiration in ascending steep mountain sides. Tea made from the leaves has much the taste of green tea, and if taken at night is much more effective in keeping people awake. Applied externally, Coca moderates the rheumatic pains caused by cold, and cures headaches. When used to excess, it is like everything else, prejudicial to the health, yet of all the narcotics used by man Coca is the least injurious and the most soothing and invigorating. I chewed Coca, not constantly, but frequency, from the day of my departure from Sandia, and besides the agreeable soothing feeling it produced, I found that I could endure long abstinence from food with less inconvenience than I should otherwise have felt, and it enabled me to ascend precipitous mountain sides with a feeling of lightness and elasticity and without losing breath. This latter quality ought to recommend its use to members of the Alpine Club, and to walking tourists in general. To the*

*Peruvian Indian Coca is a solace which is easily procured, which affords great enjoyment and which has a most beneficial effect. The shepherd watching his flock has no other nourishment."*

But just as the mass of Peruvian manuscript in Spanish and native Quichua was of little utility to the working world until rendered so by the practical hand of the translator, so the wonderful qualities of Coca remained locked as a scientific mystery unsolvable by the multitude, until it was finally released from its enchanted spell as through some magic touch of a modern Merlin.

# Mariani

It has been said that a man is created for some especial work, and this seems happily applied in the present instance. Angel o Mariani was born in Bastia, the largest city of Corsica, where a foundation for scientific training through an ancestry of physicians and chemists preceded him. But better than ancestry is the work that a man does which shall live after him. Reared in an atmosphere where chemical possibilities were daily thoughts—while united with these was a love for books, and allied art and antiquities—it seemed but natural that he should experiment on the then much talked of Coca of the Incas, an ideal of endurance, interest in which the tales of travellers and scientists from Cieza to Mantegazza had only intensified. The problem of the elixir of life, so baffling to philosophers since long before the days of Hermes Trismegistus, which many now believed was pent up in Coca—seemed capable of as definite solution as is possible through human intervention.

*Preparations of Coca manufactured by Mariani are entirely different in aroma and action from other Coca preparations.*

Commencing investigation with the unmistakable evidence regarding the properties of Coca, it was sought to present these in a positive and available form, which fluid and solid extracts, or the volatile herb, had not uniformly preserved. Experimentation led to combining several varieties of leaf, setting aside those which contained chiefly the bitter principle—since known to be cocaine—and selecting those which contained the aromatic alkaloids. An extract of these blended leaves embodied in a wholesome wine, was found to represent the peculiar virtue of Coca as so much prized by the native users.

There is no secret other than method claimed in the process which has made the name of its inventor synonymous with that of Coca, though I heard an anecdote related of this gentleman—who personally scrutinizes every detail of manufacture, that: "after everything else is done he goes around and drops something else in." Whether this be so or not, it is certain that the preparations of Coca manufactured by Mariani are entirely different in aroma and action from other Coca preparations which I have examined. These latter have not the agreeable flavor of Coca, but the fluid extracts are usually bitter and the wines have a peculiar birchlike taste comparable with the smell of an imitation Russia leather. That this "musty cellar flavor," as it is technically termed, is due to the quality of Coca leaf was evidenced by a preparation of wine made for me in Paris in the fall of 1898, from choice leaves direct from the Caravaya district, which, however, were rich in cocaine.

## A Coca Savant

It seems appropriate in a history of Coca that I should say something of the personality of one whose life work has been devoted to rendering the "divine herb" popular. It may be said that Coca is the hobby of Mariani. It is his recreation, his relaxation and constant source of pleasure,

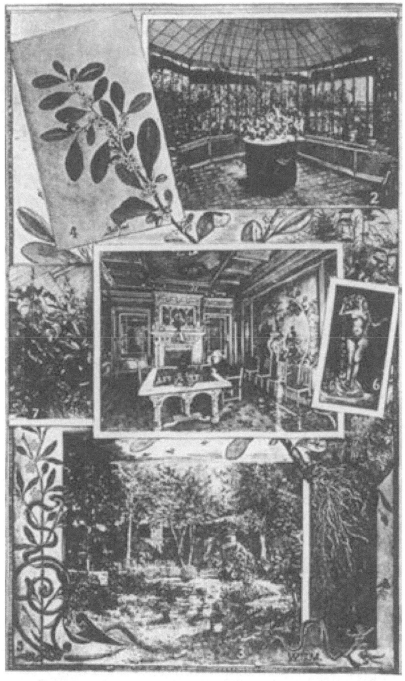

*Mariani's Coca Garden*

wholly removed from sordid commercial interests. At
Neuilly, on the Seine, Paris, France, where his laboratory is
located, his study is tastefully arranged with rich tapestries
and carvings, in which the exquisite designs possible from
conventionalizing the Coca leaf and flower are so artistical-
ly used as the motif of decoration that they are not obtru-
sive but must be pointed oat in order to be recognized.
Here he has extensive conservatories, which are filled with
thousands of Coca plants of various species, among which
he takes the greatest delight in experimenting upon peculiarities of growth and cultivation. From this collection
specimen plants have been freely distributed to botanical
gardens in all parts of the world.

As I had difficulty in preserving appropriate examples
of the Peruvian shrub for my study, ten choice Coca plants
were sent to me from Neuilly, and these, for proper care
and preservation, I presented to the New York Botanical
Garden, while still being permitted to continue my experiments upon them. In addition to this courtesy, I have been
the recipient of numerous favors from M. Mariani, who has
generously accorded me details upon the subject of research not readily obtainable elsewhere, and who literally
extended the resources of his vast establishment to the furtherance of my investigation. Aside from papers in current
journals Mariani wrote a monograph upon Coca and its
therapeutic application, a translation of which by Mr. J. N.
Jaros, of this city, has been the most available authority for
the English reader.

I am convinced no more happy realization can occur to
this savant than the knowledge that his efforts to render
Coca popular and available have met with a spontaneous
approval from representative personages in various parts
of the world. Entirely aside from any personal interest,
a voluminous testimony has literally showered in from
those whose motive and sincerity must be accepted as an
unquestionable regard for recognized merit. Eminent art-

ists and sculptors have painted and chiseled some dainty examples which serve to typify their esteem for a modern elixir vita? Roty, President of the *Academie des Beaux Arts,* and probably the most eminent living medalist, has executed a presentation medal of appreciation. Famous musical composers, such as Gounod, Faure, Ambrose Thomas, Massenet, and many others have sung their hosannas in unique bars of manuscript melody. Poets and writers without number have versed the qualities of the Coca leaf and the present happy idealization of its powers. Royalty has set upon it the meritorious seal of patronage, and the modern Church, more liberal than its edicts of long ago, has welcomed its use. Only recently Pope Leo XIII sent a golden medal of his ecclesiastical approval, for it is said that for years His Holiness has been supported in his ascetic retirement by a preparation of Mariani's Coca, of which a flask constantly worn is, like the widow's cruse, never empty.

So numerous have been these expressions from eminent characters of the day, that it has been possible to compile from them a cyclopedia of contemporary biography which has already reached several large octavo volumes. A brief outline of each notable is given, with an etched portrait, and often accompanied by a sketch showing some known forte of the individual. Where these are artists their impromptu illustrations display a happy humor associated with their characteristic touch.

The resultant compilations, exquisitely printed and bound as an *edition de luxe,* are much sought by bibliophiles. A short time since, while the Princess of Battenberg was on a visit at Nice, she was presented with one of these copies, and in acknowledging the courtesy suggested that her mother, the Queen of England, would be delighted to have one for her private library. In fulfillment of such a hint, which was accepted as an imperial command, two sets, especially illuminated by Atalaya, were forwarded to Her Majesty, who wrote that she considered them among the finest specimens in her collection.

"With this first advance in securing the properties of the leaf in convenient form for use, came the important researches of Niemann upon the alkaloids of the Coca leaf. The work of this investigator was speedily followed by a host of ardent experimenters, as is recounted in the chapter which relates some of the chemical problems involved in Coca. The more pronounced advantages, however, which were to benefit all humanity, were not immediately utilized, and for nearly a generation cocaine was regarded as but an expensive curiosity of the laboratory.

In 1884 the attention of the scientific world was suddenly concentrated on the remarkable possibilities of the Coca leaf through the discoveries of Dr. Carl Koller, on the application of cocaine to the surgery of the eye. Manufacturing chemists turned their attention to the parent plant, for there was a desire to make the product now brought so prominently into great demand as to be held at exorbitant prices. An incident will serve to illustrate its rarity at that time. I was then on the staff of physicians at the hospitals of the almshouse, Black-well's Island, and through a former interest as a pharmacist in the study of Coca, was desirous of obtaining some of the new alkaloid. Upon requisition a supply of about a drachm of a two per cent, solution of cocaine was sent for use in a service of some two thousand patients.

Among my classmates, in the medical department of the University of the City of "New York, was my friend Henry H. Iiusby, then regarded as a botanist of great promise, and at present Professor of Materia Medica of that university and of the New York College of Pharmacy. Immediately after his graduation he went to South America on a botanical expedition for Parke, Davis & Co., and they forwarded instructions to him to devote sufficient time to study Coca in its native home. The result of his research is full of interest as showing the similarity between modern customs of Coca cultivation, as compared with the descriptions of the early Spanish historians. These investigations were chiefly carried out in the district of Coroico, of the Yungas of Bolivia. This botanist was the first to clearly show that: "the best quality of Coca leaves, to a manufacturing chemist, means those which will yield the largest percentage of crystallizable cocaine, while the same leaf might be considered for domestic consumption as representing one of the lower grades." For, as he has explained: "The Indian selects a Coca rich in the aromatic and sweet alkaloids instead of the bitter leaf in which cocaine is predominant." Since 1885, most of the writings and the experiments of physiologists upon Coca seem to have been based upon the idea of a single active principle which should represent the potency of the leaf. As is clearly indicated in the history which has been traced through nearly four centuries, this is a false supposition. The qualities of Coca are not fully represented by any one of its alkaloids thus far isolated.

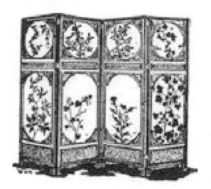

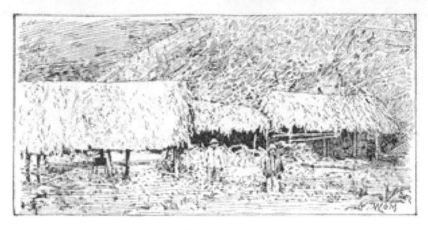

## Chapter 3

# The Botany of Coca

CA—the "divine plant" of the Incas, belongs to the family of the Erythroxylacew, which is broadly distributed . throughout the tropical world. There are two genera, the Erythroxylon and Aneulophus. Of the former there are at least a hun-prdred species, the majority of which are found in South America; in tropical Asia there are six, in Africa five or more, and two in Northern Australia. The characteristics of the entire family are similar, while several peculiarities are predominant, among which are the nerve markings of the leaf, the tongue-like appendage of the petals of the flower, and the early obliteration of a certain number of the original compartments of the fruit, two or three of these aborting even while in flower, leaving an indication of their former presence only by minute openings.

Peyritsch, in an elaborate classification of the genus Ery-throxylon, makes four divisions of this in accordance with the size of the leaf and certain peculiarities of the flower. The first division describes seven species growing in Brazil, Northern Mexico and Cuba, of which the leaves are up to a thumb's length, the flowers occurring from one to six in the axils of the bracts, or scales, the styles being at least in part free.

# Early Classification

The second division enumerates twenty-eight species, among them several employed for economic uses, E. anguifu-gum, Mart., E. squamatum, Swaitz, and E. areolatum, Jacq., together with E. Coca, Lam., which is by far the most important of the entire family. The plants of this species are scattered through Peru, Colombia, Guiana, Panama—E. Pana-maense, Turez, Mexico—E. Mexicanum, HBK., Colombia— E. cassinioides, PI. et Lind, and E. rigidulum, DC. In this division the leaves are commonly longer than the thumb, though less than a finger's length. The flowers occur from three to ten in clusters, the arrangement of the styles being as in the first division.

The third division embraces thirty-five species, found in Peru, Guiana, Colombia and Brazil. Among this is E. Pul-chrum, St. Hil., growing in the province of Rio Janeiro and locally known as subrayil or arco de pipa, and E. Sprucea-num, Peyr., growing in Panure to Rio Uaupes, the E. suhe-rosum, St. Hil., and E. tortuosum, Mart. The Mama Coca of Martius is also classed here as a distinct species. The leaves of this class are of a finger's length or over. The styles of the pistil are joined up to their stigmas.

In the fourth division there are twelve species, the leaves of all of which are from a span to a foot or more long. In the entire classification eighty-two species are described.

Many of the species of Erythroxylon are employed for economic uses. E. anguifugum is used in Brazil as a remedy against snake bite. E. campestre is employed in the same country as a purgative. The bark of E. suberosum, and also of E. tortuosum., yields a brownish red dye. The former is termed in Brazil gallinha choca and mercurio do campo.

E. areolatum is a native of the northern parts of South America and Jamaica, in the latter place being known as red wood, or iron wood, and some excellent timber is derived from this species. It is a small tree from fifteen to

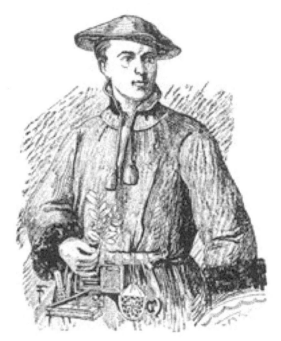

*Botanist Linnaius in Early Life*

eighteen feet in height, with a trunk from five to six inches in diameter, growing in the lowlands. The twigs and leaves of this species are said to be refrigerant and when mixed with benne oil form a refreshing liniment, while the bark is also a tonic and the sub-acid of its fruit is purgative and diuretic. The wood of E. hyperici folium is the Bois d'kuile of the Isle of France. E. monogynum is a native of the East Indies, where it is known under the native name of gadara. Its wood is fragrant and takes a beautiful polish, being considered as a sort of bastard sandal. An empyreumatic oil is derived from it, which is used in preserving the wood of the native boats. The important properties of Coca have directed attention to the plants of these several species of the Erythroxylon family in the hope that their leaves might contain a similar series of alkaloids.

## Characteristics of Coca

The first attempt at any technical description of Coca was that made by Monardes some years after the early publications upon the conquest of Peru. The earliest purely botanical classification appears to be that of Plukenet, in 1692. He describes the "Mamacoca," or the "Mother of Coca," as the deified name used among the Peruvians. About a genera¬tion later Antoine de Jussieu described the specimens which he had received from his broth¬er Joseph while he was with the expedition of La Conda-mine. Jussieu placed Coca in the family of the Malpighiacem of the genus Setfaia because of certain characteristics of the leaf and the three-compartment fruit.

Cavanilles, who drew his account and his illustrations of the plant from these examples, which were pre¬served in the herbarium of the Museum of Natural History at Paris, also followed this classification.

Dr. Browne in 1756, in his Natural History of Jamaica, included Coca among the plants of that region and placed it in the family Erytliroxylwn, de-

CARL VON LINNE. [Linnæus.]

riving this generic name from the red color of the wood of some local species. About this same time Linna;us placed Coca in the family of the Erythroxylece of the genus Erythroxylon, and subsequently this classification was followed by Antoine Laurent de Jussieu, a nephew of Joseph, who changed the classification from Malpighiads because of certain characteristics of the Coca flower.

The observation was made by the poet Goethe in his "Metamorphosis of Plants," that the flower was merely a

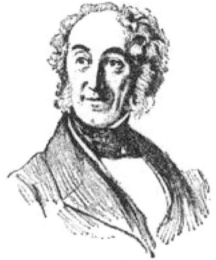

reproduction of the modified plant leaf, just as the stem, trunk, stalk or root is shaped to satisfy particular requirements, all originating from the germinal embryo in the seed. Because it determines the perpetuation of the plant, botanists regard the flower as an important organ in the consideration of any classification.

Sir W. J. Hooker.

The Erythroxylons differ from the Malpighiads by their flowers growing from amongst small imbricated scales, having no glands on the calyx, capitate stigmas, and having the ovules united superiorly. Lamarck has followed the classifi¬cation of Antoine Laurent de Jussieu, and this has since been regarded by the majority of authorities as classic. Eichler and Martius have continued the description of the early Jussieu, while Ballieu, Planchon, and Bentham and Hooker, because of the frequent occurrence of a five-compartment fruit, have placed Coca with the Linacew—the flax family, and have assigned it as number thirty-four of the division of that order. Commers has placed Coca in the genus Venelia and Roelana, and Spreng associates it with the Steudelia, while Humboldt, Bon-

pland and Kunth class it with Sethia, of which Jussieu formed
a genus.

One of the most marked characteristics of the Coca leaf
is the areolated portion bounded by two longitudinal elliptical lines curving toward the midrib. These lines are commonly more conspicuous on the under surface of the leaf.
The areolated portion is slightly concave, and of a deeper
color than the rest of the leaf, probably from a closer venation. This peculiarity is not confined to the Erythroxlon
Coca. It is marked in E. areolatum, and it furnishes a character for the section Areolata of de Candolle's Prodromus,
Vol. I, p. 575, in which five specimens are included. In
many other species, where there are no dcmarking lines,
the leaves are sometimes marked by similar bud pleatings
or have a peculiar color bounding the area. In his early account of this species Browne described the leaf as: "Marked
with two slender longitudinal lines upon the back which
were the utmost limits of that part of the leaf which was
exposed while it lay in a folded state."

Some botanists have considered the characteristic
lateral lines of the Coca leaf as nerves. Martius was of the
opinion these result from pressure of the margin of the
leaf as it is rolled toward the midrib while in the bud, the
pinching of the tissue causing the substance of the leaf
to be raised, resembling a delicate nerve. The lines have
been designated as "tissue folds," but there is no fold in
either the epidermis or substance of the leaf. Histologically
the lines are formed by a narrow band of elongated cells,
which resemble the collenchyma cells of the neighboring
epidermis, and these doubtless serve to stiffen the blade.
The lines have no connection wjth the veins of the leaf and
in transmitted light seem like mere ghostly shadows which
vanish under closer search.

Many observers have supposed they had found the
original locality of wild Coca. Alcide d'Orbigny describes

in his travels, having entered a valley covered with what
he sup¬posed to be the wild Coca shrub, but thinking he
might be mistaken, he showed the plant to his mule driv-
er, who was the proprietor of a cocal in Yungas, and he
pronounced it undoubtedly Coca and gathered a quantity
of the leaves.8 It has been asserted that wild Coca may be
found in the province of Cochero, and one of the former
governors of Oran, in the province of Salta, on the northern
borders of the Argentine Republic, claims to have found
wild Coca of excellent quality in the forests of that district
Poeppig also described having found wild specimens,
known by the natives as Mama Coca, in the Cerro San
Cristobal, near the Huallaga, some miles below Huanuco.
These examples closely resemble the shrubs of cultivated
Coca collected by Martius in the neighborhood of Ega, Brazil, near the borders of the Amazon, and correspond to the
wild specimens commonly found throughout Peru.

# Habitat of Coca

In Colombia Humboldt, Bonpland and Kunth described
Erythroxylon Ilondcnse as the possible type of the originally cultivated Coca shrub, but there is a difference between
the leaves of E. Coca and E. Ilondcnse in the arrangement
of their nervures, from which Pyrame de Candolle considers them as entirely distinct species. Andre speaks of Coca
in the valley of the river Cauca as in abundance in both the
wild and half-wild state, but an excellent authority denies
that Coca is found wild in Colombia.

The exact locality where Coca is indigenous in a wild
state has, however, never been determined. Though there
are many  Coca plants growing throughout the montana
outside of cultivation, it is presumed that these are examples where the seeds of the plant have either been uninten-
tionally scattered or else are the remains of some neglected
plantation where might have flourished a vigorous cocal

under the Spanish reign. There are evidences of these scattered shrubs throughout the entire region where Coca will
grow, but there is no historical data to base a conclusion
that these represent wild plants of any distinct original variety, while the weight of testimony indicates that they are
examples of the traditional plant which have escaped from
cultivation.

Although the heart of the habitat of Coca is in the Peruvian montana from 7° S., north for some ten degrees, the
shrubs are found scattered along the entire eastern curve
of the Andes, from the Straits of Magellan to the borders
of the Caribbean Sea, in the moist and warm slopes of the
mountains, at an elevation from 1,500 to 5,000 and even
6,000 feet, being cultivated at a higher altitude through
Bolivia than in Peru. Throughout this extent there are to
be seen large plantations and many smaller patches where
Coca is raised in a small way by Indians who come three
or four times a year to look after their crop. In some localities, through many miles, these cocals cover the sides of the

mountains for thousands of
feet. During the Incan period
the centre of this industry
was about the royal city of
Cuzco, and at present the
provinces of Caravaya and
of Sandia, east of Cuzco, are
the site of the finest variety
of Peruvian grown Coca. In
this same region there grows
coffee, cacao, cascarilla, potatoes, maize, the sugar cane,

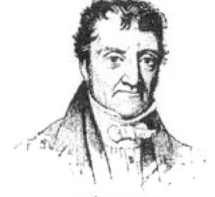

AIMÉ BONPLAND.

bananas, peaches, oranges, paltas, and a host of luscious
fruits and many valuable dyes and woods.

There are still important Coca regions about Cuzco,
and at Paucartambo and in several Indian towns along the
Huanuco valley, situated in the very heart of the northern

montana and noted for its coffee plantations. At one time
this region was accredited with supplying Coca for all
Peru, which probably meant the mining centres of Huan-
cavelica—formerly more prominent than at present—and
Cerro de Pasco, where the mines are still extensively
worked. There are fine cocals at Mayro, on the Zuzu River,
and at Pozuso—which are German colonies; at the latter
place is located the laboratory of Kitz, one of the largest
manufacturers of crude cocaine, whose product supplies
some of the important German chemical houses. Still further to the northwest—in Colombia, there are a number
of small plantations along the valley of Yupa, at the foot
of the chain of mountains which separates the province of
Santa Marta de Maracaibo, at the mouth of the Magdalena
River. Eastward from the montana Coca is cultivated near
many of the tributaries of the Amazon, and through some
portions of Brazil, where it is known as ypadil (E. Pul-
chrum, St. Ilil.). The Amazonian plant is not only modified
in appearance, but the alkaloidal yield is inferior.

## Essentials for Culture

The temperature in which Coca is grown must be equable,
of about 18° C. (64.4° F.). If the mean exceeds 20° C. (68°
F.), the plant loses strength and the leaf assumes a dryness
which always indicates that it is grown in too warm a
situation, and though the leaves may be more prolific, they
have not the delicate aroma of choice Coca. It is for the
purpose of securing uniform temperature and appropriate
drainage that Coca by preference is grown at an altitude
above the intense heat of the valleys, and where it is virtually one season throughout the year, the only change
being between the hot sun or the profuse rains of the
tropical montana. As the temperature lowers with increase
of altitude, when too great a height is reached the shrub is
less thrifty and develops a small leaf of little market value,

while as only one harvest is possible the expense of cultivation is too great to prove profitable. Even close to the equator, in the higher elevations, there is always danger from frost, and for this reason some of the cocals about Huanuco have at times suffered serious loss. All attempts at Coca cultivation on a profitable scale near to Lima have failed not only because of the absence of rain, but be-cause the season's changing is unsuited.

A peculiar earth is required for the most favorable cultivation of Coca, one rich in mineral matter, yet free from limestone, which is so detrimental that even when it is in the substratum of a vegetable soil the shrub grown over it will be stunted and the foliage scanty. While the young Coca plants may thrive best in a light, porous soil, such as that in the warmer valleys, the full grown shrub yields a better quality of leaf when grown in clay. The red clay, common in the tropical Andes, is formed by a union of organic acids with the inorganic bases of alkaline earths, and oxides—chiefly of iron—which in a soluble form are brought to the surface by capillarity. These elements enter the Coca shrub in solution through its multiple fibrous root, which looks like a veritable wig. The delicate filaments are extended in every direction to drink in moisture, and as these root-hairs enter the interspaces of the soil, the particles of wliich are covered with a film of water, absorption readily takes place. The clay soil of the montaiia affords this property in a high degree, while the hillside cultivation admits of an appropriate drainage of the interspaces without which the delicate root would soon be rotted. As the water is absorbed from the soil, a flow by capillarity takes place to that point, and so the Coca root will drain a considerable space.

It is possible a metallic soil may have some marked influence on the yield of alkaloid. At Phara, where the best Coca leaves are grown, the adjacent mountains are formed of at least two per cent, of arsenical pyrites, a fact which is

note-worthy because this is the only place in Peru where
the soil is of such a nature. Most of the soil of the Andean
hills where the best Coca is grown, originates in the decay
of the pyritifer-ous schists, which form the chief geological
feature of the sur-rounding mountains. This, commonly
mixed with organic matter and salts from the decaying
vegetation, or that of the trees burned to make a clearing,
affords what might be termed a virgin earth—terre franche
ou normale—which requires no addition of manures for
invigoration. In the conservatory it has been found, after
careful experimentation, that a mixture of leaf mould and
sand terre de bruyere, forms the best artificial soil for the
Coca plant.

Aside from an appropriate soil that is well drained,
there is another important element to the best growth of
Coca, and that is a humid atmosphere. Indeed, in the heart
of the mon-taiia it is either hazy or drizzling during some
portion of the day throughout the year, the intense glare of
the tropical sun being usually masked by banks of fog, so
that it would seem that one living here is dwelling in the
clouds. At night the atmosphere is loaded with moisture
and the temperature may be a little lower than during the
day, though there is usually but a trifling variation day
after day.

The natural life of the Coca shrub exceeds the average
life of man, yet new Cocals are being frequently set out to
re¬place those plants destroyed through accident or carelessness. The young plants are usually started in a nursery,
or alma-ciga, from seeds planted during the rainy season,
or these may be propagated from cuttings. In the conservatory slips may be successfully grown if care is taken to
retain sufficient moisture about the young plant by covering it with a bell glass. The birds are great lovers of Coca
seeds, and when these are lightly sown on the surface of
the nursery it is necessary to cover the beds at night with
cloths to guard against "picking and stealing." Before sow-

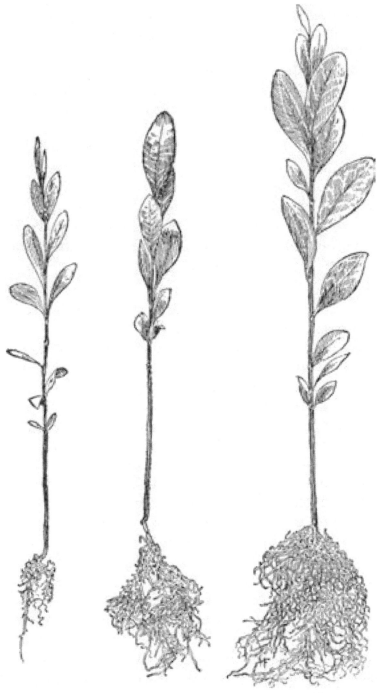

*Young Coca Plants Showing Fibrous Root*

ing the seeds are some-times germinated by keeping them in a heap three or four inches high and watering them until they sprout. They are then carefully picked apart and planted, either in hills or the seeds are simply sown on the surface of the ground, "and from that they take them up and set them in other places into earth that is well labored and tilled and made convenient to set them in." There is commonly over the beds of the nursery a thatched roof— huasichi, which serves as a protection to the tender growing shoots from the beating rain or melting fierceness of the occasional sun. The first spears are seen in a fortnight, and the plants are carefully nourished during six months, or perhaps even a year until they become strong enough to be transplanted to the field.

As a rule, all plants that are forty or fifty centimetres high (16 to 20 inches) may be set out, being "placed in rows as we might plant peas or beans." In some cases they are set in little walled beds, termed aspi, a foot square, care being taken that the roots shall penetrate straight into the ground. Each of these holes is set about with stones to prevent the surrounding earth from falling, while yet admitting a free access of air about the roots. In such a bed three or four seedlings may be planted to grow up together, a method which is the outgrowth of laziness, as the shrubs will flourish better when set out singly. Usually the plants are arranged in rows, termed uachas, which are separated by little walls of earth—umachas, at the base of which the plants are set. In some districts the bottle gourd, maize, or even coffee, is sown between these rows, so as to afford a shield for the delicate shoots against sun or rain. At first the young plants are weeded—mazi as it is termed—frequently, and in an appropriate region there is no need for artificial watering; but the Coca plant loves moisture, and forty days under irrigation will cover naked shrubs with new leaves, but the quality is not equal to those grown by natural means.

In from eighteen months to two years the first harvest, or mitta, which literally means time or season—is commenced. The leaves are considered mature when they have begun to assume a faint yellow tint, or better—when their softness is giving place to a tendency to crack or break off when bent, usually about eight days before the leaf would fall naturally. This ripe Coca leaf is termed by the Indians cacha.

# Harvest

The Coca shrub, growing out of immediate cultivation, will sometimes attain a height of about twelve feet, but for the convenience of picking, cultivated plants are kept down to less than half that height by pruning—huriar or ccuspar—at the time of harvesting, by picking off the upper twigs, which in-creases the lateral spread of the shrub. The first harvest—or rather preliminary picking, is known as quita calzon, from the Spanish quitar—to take away, and calzon—breeches. As the name indicates, it is really more of a trimming than what might be termed a harvest, and the leaves gathered at this time have less flavor than those of the regular mittas. Each of the harvests is designated by name—which may vary according to the district. The first regular one in the spring—mitta de marzo, yields the most abundantly. Then, at the end of June, there is commonly a scanty crop known as the mitta de San Juan—the harvest of the festival of St. John—while a third, following in October or November, is the mitta de Todos Santos—the harvest of all saints.

Usually the shrubs are weeded only after each harvest, and there seems to be a prejudice against doing this at other times, though if the cocals are kept clear the harvest may be anticipated by more than a fortnight. Garcilasso tells how an avaricious planter, by diligence in cultivating his Coca, got rid of two-thirds of his annual tithes in the first harvest.

Picking exerts a beneficial influence on the shrub, which otherwise would not flourish so well. The gathering—palla —is still done by women and children—palladores as they are termed—just as was the custom during the time of the Incas, though the Colombians will not permit women to take part in the Coca cultivation at any time. Many writers have spoken of the extreme care with which the leaves are picked or pinched from the shrub, one by one; but to a ca-

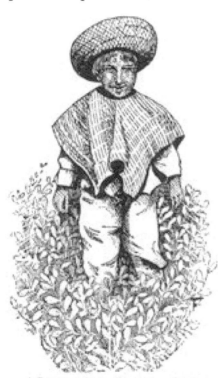

sual observer the gathering seems to be done far more carelessly. The col¬lector squats down in front of the shrub, and taking a branch strips the leaves off with both hands by a dexterous movement, while avoiding injury to the tender twigs. The pickers must be skilled in their work, for not only a certain knack, but some little force is requisite, as is shown by the wounds occa- sioned to even the hard skin of the hand of those who are accustomed to the task.

The leaves are collected in a poncho or in an apron of coarse wool, from which the green leaves—termed

A LITTLE COCA PICKER —*Brettes.*

matu—are emptied into larger sacks—materos, in which they are conveyed to the drying shed—matucancha. Four or five ex¬pert pickers in a good cocal can gather a cesta— equivalent to a bale of twenty-five pounds, in a day. Har- vesting is never commenced except when the weather is dry, for rain would immediately spoil the leaves after they have been picked, rendering them black in color and unsalable, a condition which the Indians term Coca gonupa, or yana Coca.

Coca when gathered is stored temporarily in sheds—matuhuarsi, which open into closed courts, the cachi, or matu-pampa, and the contents of these warehouses indicate the pros-perity of the master of the cocal. In the drying yards of these places the leaves are spread in thin layers two or three inches deep, either upon a slate pavement—pizarra, or simply distributed upon a hard piece of clear ground of the casa de hacienda. The closest guardianship must now be maintained over the leaves during the process of drying, and on the slightest indication of rain they are swept under cover by the attendants with the greatest rapidity. Drying may be completed within six hours in good weather, and when properly dried under such favorable conditions, the leaf is termed Coca del dia and commands the highest price.

A well-cured mature Coca leaf is olive green, pliable, clean, smooth and slightly glossy, while those which are old or are dried more slowly assume a brownish green and are less desirable. After drying, the leaves are thrown in a heap, where they remain about three days while undergoing a sort of sweating process. When this commences the leaf is crisp, but sweating renders it soft and pliable. After sweating the leaves are again sun dried for a half hour or so, and are then ready for packing. If the green leaves cannot be immediately dried, they may be preserved for a few days if care be taken not to keep them in heaps, which would induce a secondary sweating or decompo-sition and give rise to a musty odor, termed Coca ccaspada, which clings even to the preparations made from such leaves.

# Curing the Leaf

The refinement of curing maintains a certain amount of moisture in the leaf, together with the peculiar Coca aroma, and it is exact discernment in this process which preserves the delicacy of flavor. When drying has been so prolonged as to render the leaf brittle and without aroma, the quality of Coca is destroyed. It has been suggested that an improvement might be made in drying through the use of sheds, where the leaves could be exposed in layers to an artificial heat, and a current of dry air, after the manner of the secaderos used in Cuba for drying coffee. But whether because of an unwillingness to adopt new methods, or because of some peculiar influence of the atmosphere impart-

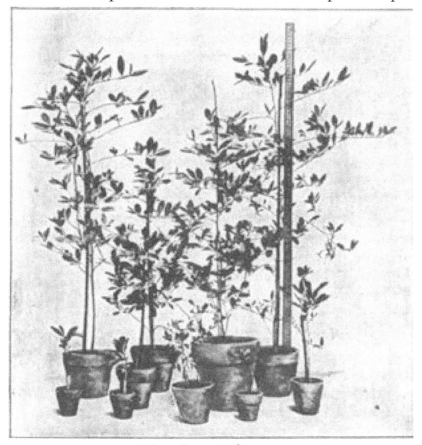

### Ten Coca Plants
The upright rule on the right is one metre high. These plants, presented to the New York Botanical Garden, have in two years fully doubled in size.

ed to the leaf in the native way of drying, all attempts to employ artificial methods have proved unsatisfactory.

The exquisite little creamy white flower of Coca is seen in the fields of the cocals after each harvest, the flowering con-tinuing for about two weeks. The Coca plants which were presented to the New York Botanical Garden have continued to blossom at irregular intervals throughout the year, while M. Mariani told me that the shrubs grown in his conservatories flower in October. The blossoms are very delicate and the petals quickly fall.

When the fruit has formed it changes color in ripening, through all the hues from a delicate greenish yellow to a deep scarlet vermilion, and upon the same shrub there may be a number of such colorations to be seen at one time. Monardes, writing centuries ago, said: "The fruit is in the form of a grape, and as the fruit of the myrtle is reddish when it is ripening, and about of the same dimensions— when attaining its highest maturity becoming darker black." I was going to say that the fruit resembles the smallest of oval cranberries, both in color and in shape, for I at one time found some little cranberries which appeared so much like the Coca fruit as to seem almost identical; but all cranberries are not alike, and there has already been too much confusion in hasty compari-son, so I shall reserve my description for the more technical details. The fruit is gathered while yet scarlet during the March harvest, but if it is permitted to remain on the bush it becomes dark brown or black and shrivels to the irregular lob-ing of the contained nut.

In selecting the seeds care is taken to cast aside all fruit that is decayed, the balance being thrown into water, and those which are light enough to float are rejected as in-dicating they have been attacked by insects. The balance are then rotted in a damp, shaded place, to extract the seed, which is washed and sun dried. When it is desired to preserve these any length of time the fruit is exposed to the hot sun, which dries the fleshy portion into a protective coating. But the seeds do not keep well. In Peru perhaps they will retain germinating power for about fifteen days, while those from plants grown in the conservatory must be planted fresh, when still red, for if allowed to dry they become useless.

With every detail to cultivation which tradition has inspired, the Coca crop is not always secure, for the cocals are subject to the attacks of several pests, which, while a constant source of annoyance may at times seriously damage the shrubs. Below an altitude of four thousand feet there is the ulo, a little butterfly, which during a dry spell deposits its eggs, and as the grubs develop they devour the younger leaves. In the older cocals an insect called mougna sometimes introduces itself into the trunk of the shrub and occasions its withering. M. Grandidier speaks of a disease termed cupa, or cachupa, in the valley of the Santa Marta, which has destroyed an entire crop within eight days. From an attack of this not only the immediate leaf is rendered small and bitter, but during the following year the shrub remains unpro-ductive, and a gall-like excrescence is developed termed sarna mocllo—seeds of gall. Some cultivators at the first indica-tion of this disease prune the affected twigs and so succeed in raising a new crop by the next harvest.

# Pests

The ant, cuqui, which is a great pest through all the mon-taiia, is a dangerous evil to the Coca plant. It not only cuts the roots, but disintegrates the bark and destroys the leaves, and in a single night may ruin an entire plantation. In fact, the sagacity of the traditional ant is outdone by these pests. Some of them are capable of carrying a kernel of corn, and an army of them will run off with a bag of corn in a night, kernel by kernel, making a distinct trail in the line of their depredations. They build their nests of leaves, twigs and earth, and even construct an underground system of channels to sup-ply their hillocks with water. It is extremely difficult to keep them out of a cocal, as they will burrow under the deepest ditches, and the only method of being free from them is to destroy their hills wherever they are found. Another enemy to the shrub is a long bluish earthworm, which eats the roots and so occasions the death of the plant. Then a peculiar fungus, known as taja, forms at times on the tender twigs, occasioned by injury or from poor nutrition. Aside from these pests, there are a number of weeds which are particularly injurious to Coca, among which are the Panicum platicaule, P. scandens,

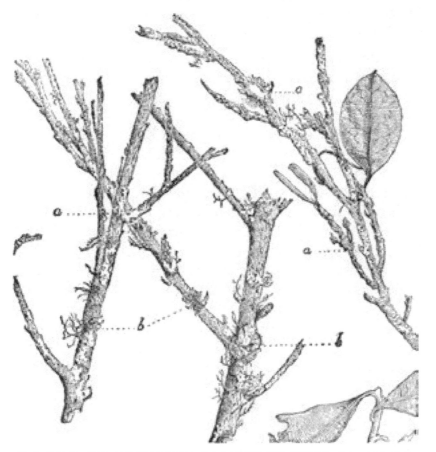

*LACCO OR LICHENS ON SPECIMENS OF COCA.*

P. decumbens, Pannisctum Peruvianum, Drimaria, and
Pieris arachnoidea." These plants grow rapidly and take so
much nourishment from the soil as to destroy the nutrition
of the Coca shrub. For a similar reason the planting of anything between the rows is now abandoned.

There grows on the trunks and branches of the older Coca shrubs various species of lichens, termed Iacco,
which, while not known to be detrimental, may even have
a marked in-fluence on the alkaloidal yield of the leaf. Two
very pretty specimens in the herbarium of Columbia University show the Parmelia and Usnea. These formed part
of a collection made by Miguel Bang, during 1890, in the
Province of Yun-gas, Bolivia, from a cocal at an altitude of
6,000 feet.

In describing any plant it is the ideal of botanists to
base their studies upon an example growing under natural
con-ditions. It is inferred that cultivation causes a variabil-
ity which may occasion considerable alteration from the
original type. Considering the centuries elapsed during
which we have any historical references to the use of Coca
among the Peruvians, it is remarkable to note how uniformly the characteristics of the plant are continued. Even
at the period of the Spanish invasion there was a tradition which traced its revered use among the Incans back
through many centuries, when it was employed for the
precise purposes for which it has been continued. Yet for
hundreds of years after the first facts concerning Coca were
introduced into Europe the available knowledge was largely legendary, and because of the phe¬nomenal properties
always assigned to its use Coca was commonly regarded
as fabulous. During all this period, however, the plant has
maintained its classic peculiarities, and supposed variations probably result more from the demands of commerce
than through a natural modification.

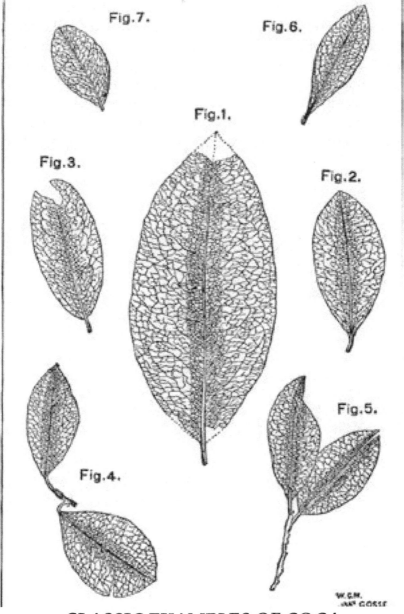

## *CLASSIC EXAMPLES OF COCA,*

1. E. Coca of Commerce.   2. K. Coca, Bonpiand : (Cuzco).   3.
E. Coca, Weddle; (Bolivia).   4. E. Coca, Toeppig: (Peru).   5. E.
Coca, Triana ; (New Granada).   C. B. Coca, Triana;  (New Grana-
da).   7. E. Coca, Ilondense, Knnth:  (New Granada).

In studying the history of a plant it would seem the proper course should be to endeavor to first trace its tradi¬tional description and uses and to then harmonize these with modern scientific facts. Unfortunately in the case of Coca, the earlier records have been largely ignored through prejudice, the descriptions which have been presented to the scientific world having often been the arbitrary outcroppings of convenience based upon the writings of travellers

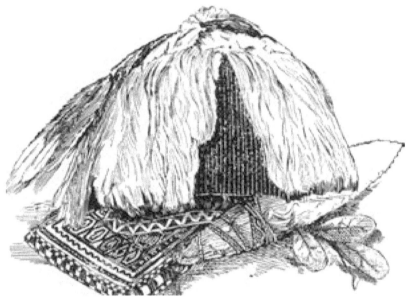

*Feather Cap & Flint Knife From Ancient Peruvian Mummy Pack.*

through certain localities, while the conclusions drawn from these accounts have been of a generalizing nature. It seems only necessary to suggest this possible source of error to show how readily confusion may be engendered.

It is always difficult to determine whether a plant, apparently growing wild, is a representative indigenous species which has existed from an early period or has been introduced from some distant locality. The scattering of

seeds, by the winds, or birds, as well as by other uncon-
scious means, may be one source of distribution of a plant
through a wide region, though as a rule the abode of each
species may be regarded as nearly constant. One of the
strongest evidences of the antiquity of a plant in its native
home is the finding of its fossil remains. While we have no
such record in the history of Coca, we have innumerable
examples of Coca leaves found in relics and with mummies
of great antiquity, which indicate in the strongest possible
way that Coca has been indigenous to Peru through many
hundreds of years.

Through the courtesy of the Curator of the Department
of Peruvian Antiquities at the American Museum of Natural History, I obtained a specimen of very ancient Coca
leaves, together with a little bag of llipta, all of which was
contained in a cliuspa of the ordinary Incan order. These
had been taken from a mummy pack found in a tomb at
Arica. This mummy wore a cap shaped like a Turkish fez,
woven of coarse wool in unique design, over which was a
covering of feathers, surmounted with a green tassel-like
feather, making a very imposing head dress and indicating
that the subject had been a person of rank. One hand bore
a white flint knife, with a handle made by binding cloth
about one end of the flint.

In the pack with the mummy, which had every evidence of extreme antiquity, was a papal bull dated 1571.
Allowing some twenty years for this document to have
found its way to Peru, this would make the mummy over
three hundred years old. That this was so, may be inferred
from the fact that no other European object was found in
the pack, everything being of an aboriginal order before
the influence of the Conquest had been manifest. The
leaves were dry and very brittle and of a light brownish
color. The llipta was in soft yellow lumps. A reproduction
of these leaves proves them to be of the variety which we
to-day understand as Truxillo or Peruvian Coca. They vary

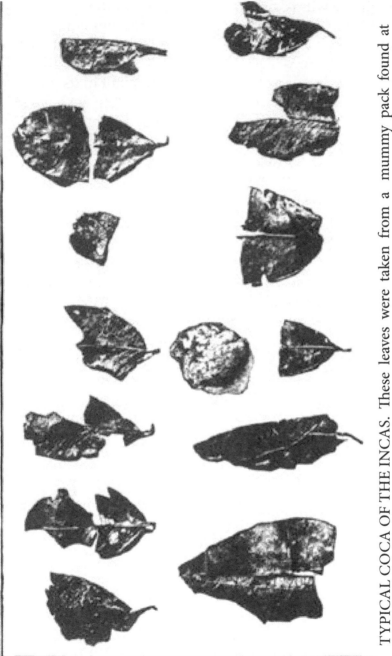

TYPICAL COCA OF THE INCAS. These leaves were taken from a mummy pack found at Arica, Peru, and presumed to be at least three hundred years old. The substance in the centre of the Illustration is a lump of Ilipta. [Compare with type of Modern Coca on opposite page.]

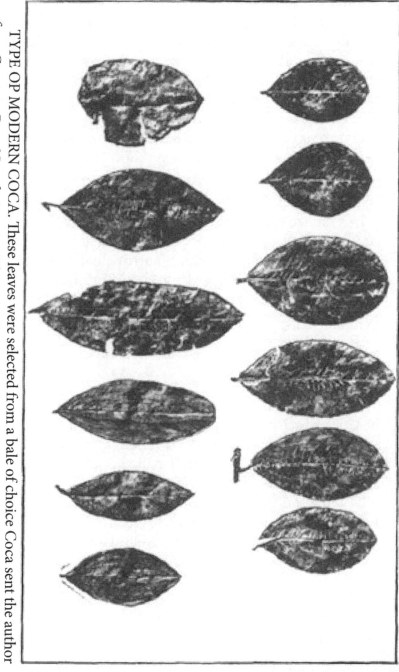

TYPE OP MODERN COCA. These leaves were selected from a bale of choice Coca sent the author from Caravaya, Peru. Note their various shapes and sizes and similarity to the ancient leaves on opposite page.

in size from a half inch in length to pieces showing a probable length of some three inches. They all plainly show the
peculiar characteristic markings of Coca, the lateral lines
being well made out. Unfortunately this mummy pack had
been treated with antiseptics before it was opened, which
rendered it impossible to note the taste of the leaves, and
there was not sufficient of them to attempt an assay. By
a comparison of the plate with the accompanying one of
recent Coca leaves it will be seen that there is no ma¬terial
difference, and certainly no ground to presume that the
classic Coca of Peru is extinct or modified.

In a choice collection of leaves from the district of
Caravaya I have found every variety of leaf present, the
pro¬nounced obovate, the long narrow leaf, the leaf with
the little point extending as though a continuation of the
inner leaf, and the distinctly lanceolate, so that it is quite
probable that more than one variety of Coca is grown in
one plantation.

# Varieties of Coca

The Coca which comes to the markets of the commercial
world is broadly grouped in two varieties, the Bolivian or
Huanuco and the Peruvian or Truxillo variety, the charac-
ter¬istic difference between the two varieties being that the
Boliv¬ian leaf is thick, dark green colored above and yellowish be¬neath, while the Peruvian leaf is smaller, more delicate,
lighter color and grayish beneath. Manufacturers of cocaine
use practically nothing except the Bolivian or Huanuco Coca,
which contains the highest percentage of cocaine and the least
quantity of associate alkaloids, which cocaine manufacturers
have regarded as "objectionable" because they will not crys-
talliz. While medicinally the Coca yielding a combination
of alkaloids is preferred, the two varieties of leaf are entirely
distinct as to flavor, being more pronouncedly bitter in proportion to the relative amount of cocaine present.

Botanists have endeavored to still further divide the com-mercial varieties of Coca because of certain peculiarities of the leaf. Some years ago Mr. Morris, of Kew, in describing the Truxillo variety of Peruvian Coca, named it Novo Grana-tense, because it was presumably a native of New Grenada. Shortly after Dr. Burck, of Buitenzorg, Java, described the variety collected by Dr. Spruce on the banks of the Rio Negro, which he named after its discoverer, E. Spruceanum. He also described a variety of Huanuco Coca which he considered approached the classic type of Lamarck, and named it Erythroxylon Bolivianum. Thus we have Peruvian or Truxillo Coca, variety Novo Granatense, Morris, and Bolivian or Huanuco Coca, which is identical with Erythroxylon Bolivianum, Burck.

The shape of the Coca leaf is a question which has excited considerable discussion among botanists, who have regarded as striking characteristics details which are seemingly unimportant to the casual observer. Undoubtedly much of the early confusion in attempts at classifying Coca from the accounts of travellers and writers has arisen from unscientific description. The illustrations have often been carelessly drawn, and this pictorial difference has represented technical faults of the illustrator rather than any actual variation of the leaf itself. In many instances the characteristics of Coca have not been clearly indicated. The result has been to con¬fuse those seeking details.

As a matter of fact, there is considerable variation in size and shape of the Coca leaf, a variation not due to the fact that the leaves have been collected from several varieties of Coca or even from several different shrubs, but upon one Coca plant there may be found leaves of varying form and size.

The Coca collected by Jussieu was from the Yungas of Bolivia, while the bulk of Coca used by the Andeans is grown in Peru. It is the plant used by these Indians, the properties of which have been exalted from the time of the Incas, to which all the traditions of Coca are attached, and really one would be more justified in saying that the specimens sent by Jussieu from Bolivia were a modification of the historical Incan plant than to say that the Peruvian grown species is a variation. The Indians prefer Peruvian Coca, and but for the importance to Bolivian Coca through cocaine less of the latter variety would be grown. Any attempt to describe Coca as a whole from any one variety, it will be seen, must be con-fusional, Bolivian Coca being

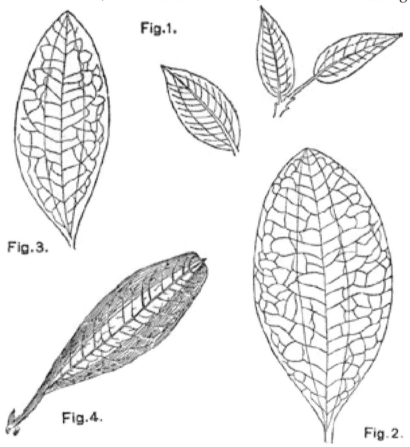

TYPES OF COCA ACCORDING TO DR. BURCK.
Fig. 1.  E. Coca, Lamarck.  Fig. 2.   B  Coca, Lam., var. BoU-vianum, Burck. Fig. 3.   10. Coca, Lam., var. Spruceanum, Burck.   Fig. 4.   E. Coca, Lam., var. Novo-Granatense, Morris.

rich in cocaine, while Peruvian Coca is richer in aromatic alkaloids. This variation is still maintained in the plants grown artificially at Paris and in the East.

Plants and seeds of several varieties of Coca have been distributed to the botanical gardens of the English colonies at Demerara, Ceylon, Darjeeling, and Alipore, where they are cultivated in a commercial way and where they have been carefully studied under the new conditions of environment. Having in mind the history of cinchona, which had been taken from its native home in the montana of Peru and so successfully cultivated in the East, it seems a natural inference that Coca may also be grown scientifically under similar facilities where the possibility for distribution would be superior to the crude Andean methods. Certain parts of Java are particularly suggestive of the Coca region of Peru. The country is traversed by two chains of mountains which are volcanic, and, as in the Andean region, the vegetation varies with the altitude. From the seaboard to an elevation of 2,000 feet the growth is of a tropical nature, and rice, cotton and spices abound. Above this to 4,500 feet coffee, tea and sugar are raised, while still higher, to 7,500 feet, only the plants of a temperate region can be grown.

There are many details essential in the cultivation of tea and coffee which suggest similar necessities in the cultivation of Coca. In Ceylon the best coffee is grown from 3,000 to 4,500 feet above the sea, where rain is frequent and the temperature moderate, and, like Coca, the higher the altitude in which the shrub can be cultivated without frost, the better is the quality of the product. Although the yield may be less, the aromatic principles are more abundant and finer than that produced in the lowlands. Similar hilly ground where there is good drainage is best adapted for the growth of tea. The shrubs do not yield leaves fit for picking before the third year, the produce increasing yearly

256                              *HISTORY OF COCA.*

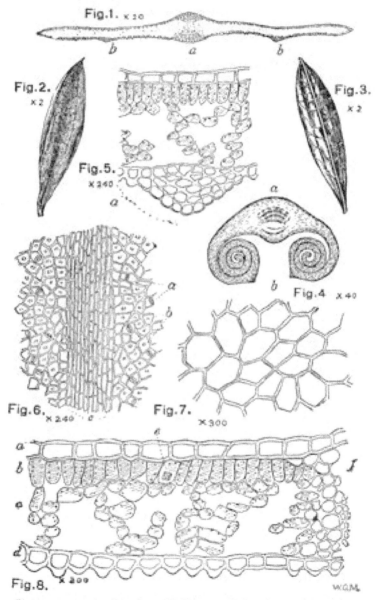

STRUCTURE OF THE COCA LEAF IN DETAIL.—*Studies Drawn from Nature.*
[See description on opposite page.]

until the tenth year. The yield from the tea plant is about the same as that from Coca, but the young leaves of tea are usually gathered, while only the matured leaves of Coca are picked.

# Stimulant

The climate, the environment, the method of cultivation and even the uses all seem paralleled in tea, coffee and Coca, but the benefits of application are immensely in favor of Coca. Tea and coffee were introduced into Europe in the sixteenth century, about the period when we have the first historical record of Coca. They were not then popular beverages as now, and it was only after much prejudice had been overcome that they were considered necessary. As the properties of Coca become better appreciated there is every reason to suppose this substance will come into as general use in every household as a stimulant—rendering a clear head instead of the hot and congested one so apt to follow the use of coffee or tea—Coca does not impair the stomach, while it possesses the added ad¬vantage of

---

DESCRIPTION OF STRUCTURE OF THE COCA LEAF, ON OPPOSITE PAGE. Fig. 1. Transverse section of a young Coca leaf near the tip; a, midrib: 6, o, lateral lines, prominent only on under surface. Fig. 2. Upper surface of an opening Coca leaf, showing manner of its unrolling. Fig. 3. Under surface of a similar leaf. Fig. 4. Transverse section of the lower half of a young Coca leaf, showing manner in which it is rolled ; a, midrib : b, prominence of lateral lines. Fig. 5. Transverse section of Coca leaf through a lateral line, a. Fig. 6. Under epidermis of a Coca leaf along a lateral line; o, stomata or breathing places; b, papillose cells; c, cells of the lateral line. Fig. 7. Upper epidermis of the Coca leaf. Fig. 8. Transverse section of a Coca leaf near the midrib ; a, epidermal cells of upper surface ; b, single row of palisade cells, with contained chlorophy! granules: e, spongy tissue of body of leaf; d, epidermal cells of lower surface; e, crystal of oxalate of lime; f, region of the midrib.

freeing the circulation from impurities instead of, like tea
and coffee, adding additional waste products to the blood
stream, as has been suggested by Morton and by Haig.

The Coca leaf affords a most exquisite subject for his-
to-logical study. Viewed in transverse section, the flattened
cells of the upper epidermis are large, oblong and of irregular shape; their outer walls are thicker than the walls
between the cells and give the surface of the leaf a wavy
outline. Beneath this protective layer is a single row of upright cells—the palisade tissue—which are filled with chlorophyl granules. These cells have very thin walls and they
are compactly set together, diverging only at their lower
edge, where the underlying spongy tissue is less compact.
Here and there maybe found cells containing crystals of oxalate of lime. Immediately beneath the palisade row of cells
are irregularly saped and loosely united, affording many
inter-cellular spaces except where the more compact tissue
surrounds the fibro-vascular bundle, which constitutes
the veins. The epidermal cells of the lower surface of the
leaf are smaller and more uniform in size than those of the
upper epidermis. The lateral walls of the cells are straight
and their outer walls are much thicker at their central part
than their marginal joinings, thus forming a papillary
projection, which is characteristic. At intervals these cells
are interrupted by the little breathing places or stomata,
bounded on either side by modified epidermal cells that
are not papillose.

A transverse section of the leaf in the bud shows that it
is rolled from its margin toward the midrib in such a way
that the lateral lines lie close together. When such a leaf
is carefully opened the midrib may be seen to be of the
same color as the leaf, pale green, and succulent, tapering
from the petiole until it is lost in the upper third of the leaf,
while from the tip there is a terminal projection, slightly
hooked, one millimetre long and of a very much paler

green than the rest of the leaf. The margin of the upper half of the leaf shows a slight wavy outline, probably due to the more rigid venation. The lateral curved lines are distinctly marked as projections on the under surface of the leaf, which is slightly concave from the midrib to the margin on either side.

## Technical Detail

Erythroxylon Coca, as cultivated in the montaiia of the Andes, grows upon a delicate shrub, which varies according to the altitude, locality and conditions of its culture. It is com¬monly kept by pruning to a height of from three to six feet for convenience of picking. Examples which are found growing out of cultivation are commonly seen ten or twelve feet high.

The root on which the Coca shrub is dependent to imbibe the nutrition for the plant forms a loose tuft or cluster of fibres, which end in fine hair-like rootlets.

The trunk is covered with a rough bark, commonly over-grown with various species of lichens—a complex colony of algae and fungi—which apparently find favorable growth from the nature of the plant and the surrounding moist at¬mosphere. The shrub branches sparingly and these are alter¬nate, either opening straight out from the sides of the trunk or ascending slightly, at times a little forked and bearing scanty foliage, the entire arrangement being adapted to afford a large surface for light and air to favor the nutrition of the plant. The color of the twigs varies from the pale fern-like green of the scaly tips to a deeper apple green, and as the firmer stem is formed the color deepens through various tints of brown until the gray bark of the trank is reached.

The leaves are arranged as the branches—alternate, and so placed that their upper surface looks toward the apex of the stem, while the lower surface is directed away from it—dorsiventral as it is termed. The shape of all varieties of the Coca leaf tends to oblong forms, narrowing at each end, in some examples gradually, in others more abruptly, the base of the leaf tapering into a short petiole or leaf stalk. Lamarck described the Coca leaf of Jussieu as "oval pointed." The leaf of Bolivian Coca is large, elliptical, oval, broader above its middle, while the Peruvian leaf is more narrow obovate, or lanceolate. The Brazilian, the Colombian and also the Javan Coca have each a smaller leaf than either of the preceding, tending to oval, broadest in the middle, from which it tapers to the apex above and to the base below. The margin of the leaf of all varieties is without notching—entire. The apex of some varieties is depressed at the extremity of the midrib— emarginate, and there is often a little soft hooked point, as though a continuation of the midrib—mucronate.   This point is light in color in the fresh leaf, but soon withers and drops in the dried specimen.

The size of the leaf varies from two centimetres to ten cen-timetres in length (about three-quarters to four inches),

---

DESCRIPTION or STRUCTURE OF COCA FLOWER, ON OPPOSITE PAGE. Pig. 1. Flower bud, a, in axil of leaves showing the bracts, 6. Pig. 2. Section of Coca flower showing the arrangement of its parts; o, the calyx; 6, the petals; c, the stamens; d, ovary, and contained ovules, e. Fig. 3. The expanded flower. Fig. 4. Flower seen from below. Fig. 5. Flower seen from above. Fig. 6. Separate petal, showing tooth-like appendage, a. Fig. 7. Petal seen from above. Pig. 8. The tooth-like appendage of the petal seen from Its attachment. Fig. 9. Flower stripped of petals; a, anthers of stamens b; r, styles and stigmas of pistil; d, ovary; e, cupule of stamens— the urceolus xlftmineus of Martius; f, calyx. Fig. 10. Pistil, with cupule and stamens removed. Pig. 11. Diagram of fertilization, [after Darwin]; A, long styled; B, short styled; a, legitimate union; 6, 6, illegitimate union.

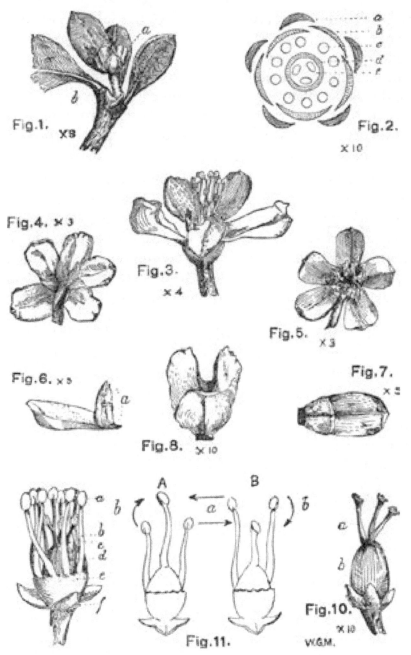

STBUCTUKE OP THE COCA PLOWER IN DETAIL—Studies
Drawn trom Mature. [See description on opposite page.]

and in breadth from two centimetres to four and one-half centi¬metres (about three-quarters to one and three-quarter inches). This variation in size is found not only in different varieties of the plant, but occurs upon different shrubs of the same variety, due to varying conditions of growth. There is, however, a variation in the size, shape and texture of the leaves upon any one shrub and even upon the same branch of one plant.

The texture of the leaf is thin, delicate and herbaceous and its substance intersected by a minute and intricate network of veins. The finer extremities of the veins as they ap¬proach the margin of the leaf anastomose like the minute apillaries of the animal circulation. By a low magnification this venation is seen to be slightly more elevated above the ventral surface or face of the leaf. Viewed by transmitted light this network appears light brown or rosy in tint, contrasting markedly with the bright green of the substance of the blade. The fresh leaf is an emerald green on the face, which is soft, smooth and even shiny, while the vinder surface is paler and grayish. The midrib is delicate and in some varieties it does not project above the face of the leaf—notably in the Javan Coca. The Bolivian Coca is

DESCRIPTION OF DETAILS OF COCA FRUIT, ON OPPO-SITE PAGE. Fig. 1. Tip of Coca spray, with ripe fruit, a, and growing stem with buds. 6. with a youug leaf and the triangular stipules at its base, c. Fig. 2. Dried fruit. Fig. 8. The six-lobed nut. Fig. 4. Longitudinal section through fruit: o, scarlet coat: 6, pink fleshy substance: c, thin shell of nut: d, white starchy-albumen : e, suspended embryo ; f, dried styles. Fig. 5. Transverse section of fruit, the references the same as in Fig. 4: g, two aborted ovules. Fig. 6. Embryo removed from seed; a, the radical : b, two cotyledons shown forced open at c. Fig. 7. a. Stamens of uniform length, seen from without the cupule, b, showing cells : c. rela¬tive size of pollen grains to anthers : d, pollen magnified 200 diameters. Fig. 8. «. Stamens of unequal length seen from within the cupule, b, showing attachment.

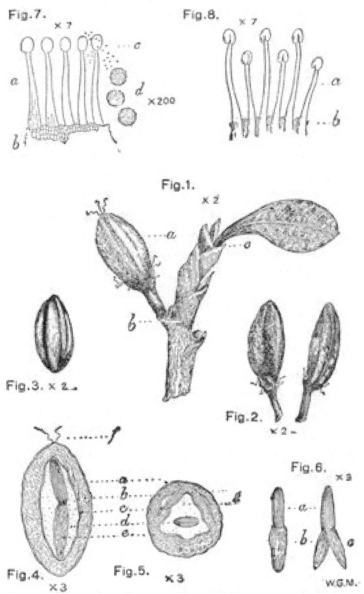

Fig.7. ×7

Fig.8. ×7

Fig.1. ×2

Fig.3. ×2

Fig.2. ×2

Fig.4. ×3

Fig.5. ×3

Fig.6. ×3

W.G.M.

DETAILS OF THE COCA FRUIT AND SEED—*Studies Drawn from Nature.*
[See description on opposite page.]

DETAILS OF THE COCA FRUIT AND SEED
Studies Drawn from Nature. [See description on opposite page.]

characterized by a ridge or crest extending along its entire upper surface, which in Truxillo Coca has been described as obliquely truncate, a feature I have not seen in any example.

To either side of the midrib there is a curved line, arranged elliptically from the petiole to the apex, presumably occasioned by the pressure of the rolled up leaf when in the bud. These lines are commonly more pronounced upon the lower surface. Gosse considers that they are more frequent in young leaves and are gradually effaced as the leaf develops, but the lateral lines are found in a majority of specimens of mature Coca leaves, and their presence constitutes a unique marking of the Erythroxylon family. By transmitted light that portion of the leaf included between the lateral line and the midrib appears of deeper shade, as though the tissue was more dense, and there is possibly a finer and more numerous division of the veins in that region. After prolonged soaking in water this deeper tint is less perceptible.

At the base of each leaf there is a pair of little appendages —stipules—ovate in shape and united along their inner borders to form a thin triangular organ, at first green with a whitish top, becoming brown and stiff, and persistent after the fall of the leaf, forming a scaly projection upon the branch.

The flower buds occur in the axils of the leaves, either solitary, or in groups of two to six. The bud is ovoid oblong, under a low power, looking very much like a bishop's mitre. As there is no definite limit to the number of leaves on a Coca shrub, so each new growth may be followed by new flowers, and it is very common to see bud, blossom and fruit upon the plant at one time. The floral plan is in five—quincunxial—the leaves of the calyx and the corolla being arranged spirally and overlapping like scales, either dextrorse or sinistrorse in the bud. At the base of the peduncle or stalk, about a centimetre long, which bears the flower, is a miniature leaf or bract. This is scaly, oval or triangular, similar to the stipules of the leaves, but shorter and more delicate.

The flowers are about a centimetre long, delicate, creamy white and exhaling a faint odor. They bear both stamens and pistils in the same blossom, and hence are termed perfect. Their outer circle of leaves—the calyx, is green, composed of five smooth, oval, triangular pointed, lobed sepals, united below and free above, the whole covered in some specimens with a delicate bloom—glaucous. That portion of the flower which is within the calyx—the corolla—is composed of five creamy leaves or petals, arranged above the sepals and alternate with them. The petals are of uniform shape, oval oblong, obtuse with a central nerve terminating in a little hooded point. Their upper surface is depressed longitudinally, which at the back shows as a keel. Their iipper two-thirds is irregularly concave and the lower third is narrowed into a triangular groove or fold. Near the base inside is an ovoid wavy tooth, or claw-like appendage, half the length of the petal, and so attached that when the petals are united to form the corolla these processes present in the centre of the ex-panded flower as a little crown. The entire corolla soon falls, leaving the naked pistil.

The flower has ten slender stamens, the filaments of which are erect, pale yellowish green, either the length of the corolla or of alternate lengths, those opposite the petals being longer than those opposite the sepals. They are inserted below the pistil, coalescing on the inner side of a short membranaceous cupule—the urceolus stamineus of Martius, which surrounds the ovary and presents obtuse tooth-like projections outside and between the filaments. Upon each filament is attached by its base a small yellow oblong compartment or anther, which contains the pollen, the grains of which are granular and spheroidal, or smooth and oval similar to those of the lily.

The pistil has three irregular, divergent cylindrical, pale yellowish, green styles, which may be either longer or shorter than the stamens. Each bears a flattened cap of loose tissue—the stigma, to receive the pollen from the opening anthers. The ovary—with its contained ovules— fertilization of which generates the seeds of the plant, is situated above the calyx. It is obovate, pale yellowish green, smooth, with three com¬partments, from the summit of each of which is suspended an ovule, but before the ovary ripens to form the fruit two of its three compartments are obliterated.

When fresh the fruit is fleshy, mucilaginous, ovate, one to one and one-half centimetres long(three-eighths to five-eighths of an inch), smooth and having the remnants of the dried styles at its apex and the adherent calyx and cupule at its base. Its color, at first pale green, changes through varying tints to scarlet at maturity and is bluish black when dried, while its form shrivels to the irregular lobed shape of the con¬tents. The seed, slightly shorter than the fruit, is pointed at each end, with six longitudinal lobes, smooth and of a pale flesh color. Its outer coat is very thin and the kernel, which completely fills the inner coat, is white, hard, albuminous and starchy. In this nutrient substance is suspended the straight green embryo or germ, half its length being the radical to form the root, while the balance composes the two flat cotyle¬dons or seed leaves, and between these is the minute plumule, from which may develop the first shoot of the new Coca plant.

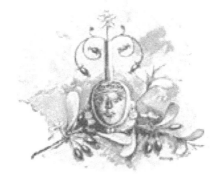

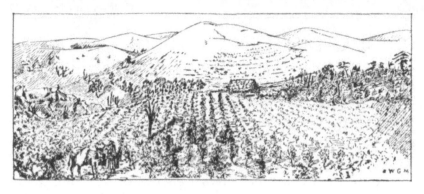

## Chapter 4

# Products of the Coca Leaf

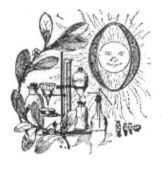

F all the problems in the study of Coca the search for the force producing qualities of the leaf is the most profound. Science, ever alert to trace with exactitude the secrets of Nature, has struggled in vain to isolate and explain this hidden source of energy. But so cleverly are the atoms associated which go to build up the molecules of power in this marvelous leaf, that though the chemist through the delicacy of analysis has from time to time placed these atoms in differing groups and thus often given to the world some new combination, the one sought element of pent up endurance inherent in Coca has remained concealed. It is like the secret of life—though known to be broadly dependent upon certain principles which may readily be explained, the knowledge of the one essential element remains as great a secret as before research began.

Though all the accounts of travellers had directed attention to the peculiar qualities of Coca in sustaining strength, at the period when the first knowledge of this leaf

reached Europe chemistry was not sufficiently advanced
to admit of an exact analysis of plant life. Indeed, science
met with little encouragement when the great powers were
engrossed in political preferment, and it was not until
the latter part of the eighteenth century that an impetus
seemed given to research after Lavoisier had laid the foundation for modern chemistry. Though he lost his life on
the guillotine through the whirligig of political fate during
the French Revolution, just as he was at the height of his
labors, a new interest was established and the work of the
French chemists became active.

## Spirit for Research

Humboldt was then making his extensive explorations
through South America, collecting data which was to serve
as a basis of research during many subsequent years. Cuvi-
er, the anatomist, was advancing his theories on the classification of animals; Fraunhofer had established a means for
studying the heavenly bodies through the spectrum, while
chemical electricity had progressed from the experiments
of Volta to the electro magnet of Ampere.

The method for expressing chemical equations, such as
are now shown by those symbolic letters and figures which
appear to the uninitiated as so many hieroglyphics, was
not understood until Dalton, in 1808, had perfected his law
of proportions. This was an important advance in chemical knowledge, for from it was built up the sign language
which in a chemical formula expresses not only the symbol
of each element, but tells the chemist the relative proportion of the combining atoms.

These fundamental facts are of interest as bearing upon
the chemical history of the Coca leaf, while the combining
nature of atoms has suggested an interesting theory that
the physiological action of a chemical medicine is influenced by its molecular weight. This has been a matter of

discussion among physiological chemists for years, and was suggested by Blake as long ago as 1841 and since by Rabuteau. Thus an element of a fixed atomic weight may have special reference to the muscular system, while another of different weight may act upon the nervous tissue, qualities which are fulfilled in the action of the several Coca bases.

Boerhaave may be said to have been the father of the present system of organic chemistry in the early part of the eighteenth century. So important were his teachings held that his works were translated into most modern languages. Al-though his attempts at analysis of living things attracted a wide interest, they could be in no manner exact, because the fundamental elements entering into the composition of all organic structure— carbon, hydrogen, oxygen and nitrogen—had not then been de¬termined. Yet so skilled were his observations, even under limited opportunities, that many of his conclusions have not since been refuted in the light of improved methods. Perhaps the earliest hint upon alkaloids was

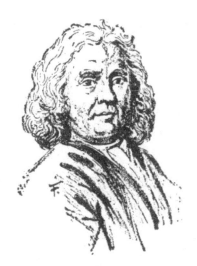

HERMANN BOERHAAVE.

that made by this scientist when he referred to the bitter principle in the juices from chewing Coca as yielding "vital strength" and a "veritable nutritive."

It was reserved for Liebig some hundred years later to perfect the science of living structures, and to show there was not that exact separation between the chemistry of the organic and inorganic world that had previously been supposed. Following the teachings of this master mind, many

compounds were constructed in the laboratory synthetically, and urea was thus produced in 1828 by Woehler, whose
name is associated with the early investigators upon cocaine. Research upon the chemistry of organic bodies was
now active. In England the work of Davy upon soils and
crops, and the investigations of Darwin, unfolded in his
theory of the origin of species, gave a new meaning to the
study of organic life.

It was but a natural outcome of this spirit for research
that turned the attention of explorers to South America,
which had remained practically a new world since its
discov¬ery. Here were to be found innumerable strange
plants in¬digenous to a country where everything was
marvelous when viewed with the comparative light of the
older world. In the height of this interest, the suggestive
hints of naturalists and travellers were incentives to further the investigations of
the European chemists.
The writings of Cieza,
Monardes, Acosta, Garci-
lasso and a host of oth-
ers upon the wonderful
qualities of the Coca leaf,
stimulated a desire to

*It was not until after
Coca had been botanically
described by Jussieu, and
classified by Lamarck, that
its chemical investigation
approached thoroughness.*

solve its tradition of ages and prove its qualities by the test
of science.

It is surprising to now look back over three centuries
and recall these early authors, to consider under what conditions they wrote, and to read with what enthusiasm and
exactness they gave expression to the knowledge they had
gained from an observation of the novel customs about
them. Thus the Jesuit father, Bias Valera, speaking of the
hidden energy of Coca, wrote: "It may be gathered how
powerful the Cuca is in its effect on the laborer, from the
fact that the Indians who use it become stronger and much
more satisfied and work all day without eating."

It was not until after Coca had been botanically described by Jussieu, and classified by Lamarck, that its chemical investigation approached thoroughness. The researches of Bergmann and Black upon "fixed air"—as carbonic acid was then termed, the discovery of hydrogen by Cavendish, of nitrogen by Rutherford and of oxygen by Priestley, each following upon the other in quick succession in the latter half of the eighteenth century, displayed the great activity of chemistry at that period. Although no result was then arrived at in the investigations upon Coca, the spirit of the time was eminently toward exactitude, and this was displayed in many endeavors to trace to a chemical principle the potency of the Coca leaf.

Attention was very naturally directed to the method in which Coca was used, and the llipta that was employed with the leaves in chewing was looked upon as having some decided influence. Dr. Unanue, who has written much concerning the customs of the Indians, was one of the first to suggest that possibly this alkaline addition to the leaf developed some new property to which the qualities of Coca might be attributed, while Humboldt, as elsewhere referred to, through an error of observation considered this added lime as the supposed property of endurance.

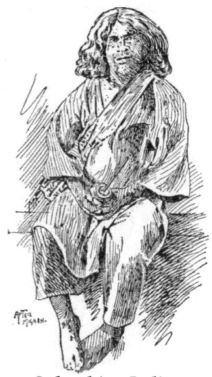

Attention had now been directed to the isolation of alkaloids from plants, and

**Columbian Indian with his Poporo**

during the first quarter of the nineteenth century several active principles were thus obtained and the possibility of tracing the hidden properties of Coca through analysis was suggested. Von Tschudi, when engaged in his extended explorations through Peru, became so impressed with the qualities of Coca that he advised Mr. Pizzi, Director of the Laboratory Botica y Drogueria Boliviano, at La Paz, to examine the leaves, which resulted in the discovery of a supposed alkaloid, but when on his return to Germany this body was shown to Woehler, it was found to be merely plaster of paris, the result of some careless manipulation.

## Early Findings

Dr. Weddell, in 1850, after a prolonged personal experience with the sustaining effects of Coca, pronounced it as yielding a stimulant action differing from that of all other excitants. This influence both he and other observers supposed might be due to the presence of theine, the active principle of tea, which had shortly before been discovered, and was that exciting considerable discussion. With this idea in view, Coca leaves were examined, and, though this substance was not found, there was obtained a peculiar body, soluble in alcohol, insoluble in ether, very bitter, and incapable of crystallization, and a tannin was obtained to which was attributed the virtues of Coca.

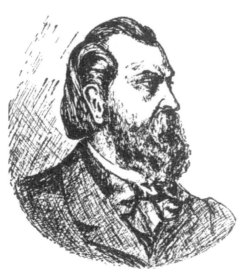

ALBERT NIEMANN.
[*From a Copper-plate Print at the Bibliothèque Nationale, Paris.*]

About this same period there was found in the leaves a peculiar volatile resinous matter of powerful odor, and two years later, from a distillation of the dry residue of an aqueous extract of Coca, an oily liquor of a smoky odor was separated together with a sublimate of small needle-like crystals, which was named "Erythroxyline", after the family of which Coca is a species. So each new investigator made a little progress, and in 1857 positive results were very nearly reached through the following process: An extract of Coca was made with acidulated alcohol, the alcohol was expelled, and the solution rendered alkaline by carbonate of soda. Upon extracting this with ether, an oily body of alkaline reaction was obtained without bitter taste, which on application to the tongue produced a slight numbness. The reaction of platinum chloride yielded with the acid solution a yellowish precipitate, soluble in water. From a distillate of the leaves with alkali there was remarked a disagreeable, strongly ammoniacal odor. Subsequently a peculiar bitter principle, extractive and chlorophyl, a substance presumed to be analogous to theine, and a salt of lime was found.

These negative findings led some to assert that Coca was inert and its properties legendary, but more careful observation has shown the true difficulty was an inability to secure appropriately preserved leaves for examination. This was made evident through an essay upon Coca by an eminent Italian neurologist, from experiences while a resident of Peru, when a host of physiological evidence emphasized the powerful nature of Coca, wholly apart from any mere delusions of fancy or superstition. The weight of facts presented proved sufficiently forcible not only to stimulate the waning spirit for scientific inquiry, but to awaken a widespread popular regard in what was now generally accepted as a plant of phenomenal nature.

In the height of this interest Dr. Scherzer, who accompanied the American frigate Novara on the expedition to

South America, opportunely brought home specimens of Coca leaves from Peru. These were sent to Professor Woehler of Gottingen for analysis, who entrusted their examinaiton to his assistant, Dr. Albert Nieman, who is regarded as the discoverer of the alkaloid cocaine. Thus this chemist entered upon the investigation of Coca not in any mere accidental way, but with an understanding of the seriousness of his research and its probable importance.

# Discovery of Cocaine

Niemann exhausted coarsely ground Coca leaves with eighty-five per cent, alcohol containing one-fiftieth of sulphuric acid; the percolate was treated with milk of lime and neutralized by sulphuric acid. The alcohol was then recovered by distillation, leaving a syrupy mass, from which resin was separated by water. The liquid then treated by carbonate of soda to precipitate alkaloid emitted an odor reminding of nicotine, and deposited a substance which was extracted by repeatedly shaking with ether, in which it was dissolved, and from which the ether was recovered by dis-tillation. There was found an alkaloid present in proportion of about one-quarter of one per cent., which was named "Cocaine," after the parent plant, and the chemical formula $C_{32}H_{2o}NO_8$, according to the old notation, was given it. Mechanically mixed with its crystals there was a yellowish brown matter of disagreeable narcotic odor, which could not be removed with animal charcoal or re-crystallization, and was only separated by repeated washings with alcohol.

Pure cocaine, as described by this investigator, is in colorless transparent prisms, inodorous, soluble in seven hundred and four parts of water at 12° C. (53.6° F.), more readily soluble in alcohol, and freely so in ether. Its solutions have an alkaline reaction, a bitter taste, promote the flow of saliva and leave a peculiar numbness, followed by a sense of cold when applied to the tongue. At 98° C. (208.4° F.) the crystals fuse and congeal again into a transparent mass, from which crystals gradually form. Heated above the fusing point, the body is discolored and decomposes, running up the

*Pure cocaine solutions have an alkaline reaction, a bitter taste, promote the flow of saliva and leave a peculiar numbness, followed by a sense of cold when applied to the tongue.*

sides of the vessel. When fused upon platinum the crystals burn with a bright flame, leaving a charcoal which burns with difficulty. The alkaloid is readily soluble in all dilute acids forming salts of a more bitter taste than the uncombined cocaine. It absorbs hydrochloric acid gas, fuses and congeals to a grayish white transparent mass which crystallizes after some days. The crystals from its solution are long, tender and radiating.

Besides cocaine, there was found in the alcoholic tincture precipitated by milk of lime a snowy white granular mass. This fused at 70° C. (158° F.), was slowly soluble in hot alcohol, more readily so in ether, and was not acted on by solutions of acids or alkalies. This substance was named Coca wax and given the empirical formula $CeeHja04$.

Upon distilling one hundred grammes of leaves, a slightly turbid distillate was obtained, which when redistilled with chloride of sodium, yielded white globular masses lighter than water and having the peculiar tea-like odor of Coca.

In the dark red filtrate from which the cocaine had been precipitated by carbonate of soda there was found after suitable treatment a Coca tannic acid, to which the formula $Ci4Hi808$ has been given.[13] This latter result, it will be remembered, was as far as Wackenroder's investigations had gone in 1853.

The atomic weight of the amorphous compound determined from the double salt with chloride of gold, was found to equal 283, and when crystallized from hot water 280, or from alcohol 288. On heating this double salt benzoic acid was sublimed from it, which was recorded as the first observation of this nature from any known alkaloid.

Following this research, the late Professor John M. Maisch of Philadelphia verified the several results. The small percentage of nitrogen announced in the original for¬mula suggested that possibly cocaine was a decomposition compound, while the nicotine odor was thought to result from a nitrogenous body or another alkaloid. To determine this, the liquor and precipitate which had been obtained by carbonate of soda were distilled over a sand bath. A syrupy liquid was left, from which the alkaloid was separated by ether, while from the distillate was collected a resin-like mass of an acrid taste, having a narcotic odor, soon lost on exposure to a damp atmosphere, while the mass became acid and was now rendered easily soluble in water and alcohol. Whether or not this principle was nitrogenous this investigator left undecided.

Continuing the same line of research as that of Niemann, and following the suggestions of Maisch, William Lossen of Gottingen carried out an extended inquiry as to the nature of cocaine, and established its formula C17H-21NO4, in accordance with the new notation. In examining its composition he found by heating it with hydrochloric acid that it was split up into benzoic acid and another body, thereby confirming the observation which had been made concerning this sublimation from the double salt of chloride of gold and cocaine. This new base he named "ecgonine," from ixyovos—son or descendant.

# Other Alkaloids

The breaking down of cocaine was subsequently shown due to hydration, by saponifying it with baryta, and also with water alone. The first change being into benzoyl-ecgonine, followed by a sublimation of benzoic acid, while from the syrupy residue the ecgonine may be separated by repeated washings with alcohol and precipitation with ether. The crystals being only dried with great difficulty.

Ecgonine, C9Hi5!S'03, crystallizes over sulphuric acid in sheaves. It has a slight bitter-sweet taste, is readily soluble in water, less so in absolute alcohol, and insoluble in ether. Heated to 198°, it melts, decomposes and becomes brown. It forms salts with the acids, most of which crystallize with difficulty. With alkalies, it forms crystallizable combinations soluble in water and alcohol. In aqueous solutions the hydro-chloride yields no precipitate with alkalies. Chloride of platinum in presence of much alcohol gives an orange yellow precipitate, chloride of mercury throwing down a yellow precipitate under the same conditions.

The unstable nature of cocaine in the presence of acids has suggested their avoidance in its preparation, plain water being considered preferable. In this process Coca leaves are digested several times at 140° to 176°, the infusions united, precipitated by acetate of lead, and filtered. The lead is removed by the addition of sulphate of soda, and the liquor concentrated in a water bath. Carbonate of soda is then added, and the whole shaken with ether to dissolve the alkaloid, when the ether may be recovered by distillation.

In his researches Lossen[17] also described the liquid alkaloid that had been hinted at by Gaedcke in 1855, and subsequently noticed by Niemann and Maisch, which, at the suggestion of Woehler,[18] who was associated in this investigation, was termed "hygrine," from vypos—liquid, to which the formula Ci2H13N was given. This was obtained by saturating the slightly alkaline mother liquor from which cocaine had been extracted with carbonate of soda and repeatedly washing with ether. Evaporation of the ethereal extract left a thick yellow oil of high boiling point with a strong alkaline reaction. Hygrine thus found is described as very volatile, distilling alone between 140° and 230° F. It is slightly soluble in water, and more readily so in alcohol, chloroform and ether, not in caustic soda, but readily in dilute hydrochloric acid. Its taste is burning and it has a peculiar odor similar to trimethylamine or quinoline. The oxalate and muriate are crystallizable, but very deliquescent.

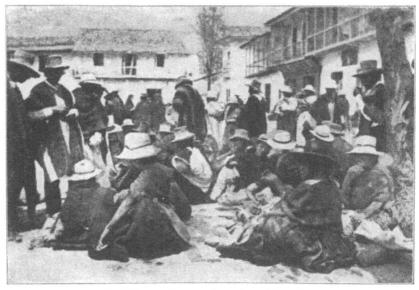

*Selling Coca in the Market*

With chloride of platinum, hygrine gives a flocculent amorphous precipitate which decomposes on heating. Bi¬chloride of mercury gives an opalescence, due to the forma¬tion of minute oily drops.

Thus far there had been found in Coca leaves a crystallizable compound of unstable composition—cocaine; a second base which was only to be crystallized with difficulty—ecgo-nine; an intermediate compound—benzoyl-ecgonine; and an oily volatile liquid of peculiar odor—hygrine; together with Coca-tannic acid, and a wax-like body. Meantime, considerable was done in a physiological way in experimenting with the new alkaloids, though little decided progress was made during the following twenty years, until 1884, when the use of cocaine in local anaesthesia was announced. The importance of this application occasioned an increased activity of investigation regarding the Coca products. This interest tended to make our knowledge of the alkaloids more exact, as well as to enrich our understanding of those inherent sustaining properties of Coca which have for past ages excited wonder.

In the early days of the cocaine industry some manufacturers asserted that the several associate substances found in Coca leaves were decomposition products, developed by changes taking place in deteriorating leaves or arising during the process of obtaining the one alkaloid. The great demand for cocaine and the high price it commanded generated an apparent unwillingness on the part of manufacturers to admit the possible presence in Coca of any other principle than cocaine. Processes innumerable were devised to force the greatest yield of alkaloid from the leaves, and some of the earlier specimens of the salt placed upon the market were more or less an uncertain mixture, dirty white in color and having a nicotine-like odor. This was defended as a peculiarity of the substance, the therapeutic action of which was asserted to be identical with cocaine, even though the appearance was not so elegant as the purer crystals. An endeavor to purify the salt by studying its sources of decomposition resulted in the separation of several important alkaloids.

The intermediate base benzoyl-ecgonine, $CioHi_{,,}NO_4$, was described as a by-product of the manufacture of cocaine, and it has been shown may be also obtained by the

evaporation of cocaine solutions. It has been prepared by
heating cocaine with from ten to twenty parts of water in a
sealed tube at 90° to 95° C, with occasional shaking until a
clear solution is obtained. This is extracted with ether to remove all traces of undecomposed cocaine, and then concentrated on a water bath and crystallized over sulphuric acid.
The crystals form as opaque prisms or needles, sparingly
soluble in cold water, more readily so in hot water, acids,
alkalies and alcohol, while insoluble in ether. It melts at 90°
to 92° C, then solidifies, and again melts at about 192° C. The
taste is bitter, its solutions are slightly acid, becoming neutral
after recrystallization. The hydrochloride, at first of a syrupy
consistency, forms tabular crystals that are freely soluble in
absolute alcohol. Mayer's reagent produces a white, curdy
precipitate; iodine in potassium iodide, a kermes brown precipitate ; chloride of gold, a bright yellow precipitate, soluble
in warm water and alcohol.

It will be recalled that Maclagan, Niemann and Maisch
had each alluded to an uncrystallizable residue in their
processes of extraction, and an effort was made to definitely determine its true quality. But just as cocaine was at first
regarded as the only alkaloid, so this amorphous substance
was studied as a whole instead of being regarded as a
mixture of bases. Coca leaves, it was asserted, contained a
crystallizable cocaine and an uncrystallizable cocaine. The
latter product has been named cocaicine, cocainoidine, and
cocamine, and is still the subject of investigation.

The relative amount of this noncrystallizable body
left in the mother liquor after the precipitation of cocaine
varies greatly and is wholly dependent upon the kind of
leaves used, or the processes to which they are subjected.
The color of Various specimens varies from dark yellow to
dark brown, while the consistence is from that of a syrupy
liquid to a sticky, tenacious solid, which, after spontaneous
evaporation, may form short, fine crystals. The odor, while
recalling nicotine, is more aromatic and less pungent; the

taste bitter and aromatic. This body is of alkaline reaction, soluble in alcohol, ether, benzole, chloroform, petroleum ether, acetic acid, etc., and of varying solubility in water, according to its consistence.

On gently heating it becomes quite fluid. It is very soluble in dilute acids, with which it forms non-crystalline salts, all of which dissolve readily in water. Dissolved in rectified spirit and treated with animal charcoal or acetate of lead, to precipitate the coloring matter, a pale yellow, sticky, non-crystalline body is obtained, which will not form crystals, even after standing for months. Solutions of the substance in alcohol, repeatedly precipitated by ammonia, yield a nearly white non-crystalline flocculent body, which is very hygroscopic, the original odor and taste remaining, no matter how often the purifying process is repeated. Evaporated at gentle heat, the solutions darken, and if evaporated to dryness the substance becomes insoluble in water. The precipitation with permanganate of potash is brownish, which, on heating, yields an odor of bitter almonds; 5 c.c. of a solution 1-1000 reduces 20 to 40 drops of a permanganate solution of the same strength.

# Controversy

Professor Stockman, of Edinburgh, made an interesting study of these mixed bases, which he originally supposed to be a solution of ordinary crystalline cocaine in hygrine, basing his conclusions on the physiological action and chemical relations. As he stated, cocaine is extremely soluble in hygrine, and once solution has occurred it is practically impossible to separate the two bodies, as they are both soluble in the same menstrua and are both precipitated by the same reagents.

This is also the case with the salts of these bodies, though not to the same extent, the presence of hygrine rendering any such samples of the salt hygroscopic, as well as imparting the peculiar nicotine-like odor of hygrine. Subsequent investigation, however, has convinced this physiologist that the substance he experimented with was cocamine dissolved in hygrine, together with some benzoyl-ecgonine.

Thus it will be seen that the earlier conclusions regarding the Coca products were erroneous from imperfect knowledge. With the increasing usefulness of cocaine this confusion is a serious matter, because these misstatements of the chemists and physiologists are often still quoted as authoritative. So positive were some of these earlier opinions that even after physiological proof showed the unmistakable presence of associate alkaloids with cocaine they were asserted, from interested motives, to be poisonous contaminations. In the face of this the result of physiological experimentation with the various Coca bases indicate that they are all more mild than cocaine, from which they differ markedly in physiological action. Dr. Bignon, Professor of Chemistry at the University of Lima, Peru, who from position and opportunities may be regarded as a competent authority upon Coca, long since asserted, when grouping the alkaloids of Coca in two classes, that the crystalline body is inodorous, while the non-crystalline has a peculiar odor and is weaker in action and less poisonous than the crystallizable cocaine.

The wholly different action of cocaine therapeutically from the Coca leaves of the Andean, or the more exact scientific preservations of Coca such as exhibited in the preparations of M. Mariani—which fully represents the action of recent Peruvian Coca, clearly indicates the presence of certain important principles in Coca, the properties of which are sufficiently distinct to markedly effect physiological action in a manner different from any one of its alkaloids. Happily we are now learning more definitely through research and experimentation, and these earlier errors are being corrected.

The diametrically opposite findings of investigators of known repute indicate that these inharmonious conclusions were not wholly the result of carelessness nor prejudice. Just as Coca experimented with by one observer repeated the traditional influence, or in some other instance proved inert, so the chemists found the result of their labors at variance. Much of this confusion was cleared away when the botanists explained that there are several varieties of Coca. Those qualities which had formerly been attributed to superstitious belief, or which when reluctantly accepted as possibly present in

*Much of this confusion was cleared away when the botanists explained that there are several varieties of Coca.*

an extremely fugitive form which was lost through volatility, were shown to be dependent upon the variety as much as upon the quality of the Coca leaf employed in the process of manufacture.

Cocamine, C10H23NO4, was originally studied in the alkaloids obtained from the small leaf variety of Coca by Hesse.[26] It was regarded by Liebermann as identical with a base which he described as y-isatropyl-cocaine, and afterward termed a truxilline, because supposedly found only in the Truxillo variety of Coca.

The research leading to these conclusions provoked bitter controversy between these two investigators. It has since been determined that cocamine is of the same empirical composition as cocaine, though weaker in anaesthetic action. It is a natural product of several varieties of Coca, particularly of that grown in Java. From hydrolysis by mineral acids cocamine yields cocaic, isococafc and homo-iso-cocaic acids, while from its isomeride there is formed in a similar way a-isotropic or fitruxillic acid. Both cocaic and iso-cocaic acids yield cinnamic acid and other products on distillation. Subsequently a similar body was prepared synthetically from ecgonine and cinnamic anhy-

dride, and named cinnamyl-cocaine. It forms large colorless
crystals, melts at 120°, is almost insoluble in water, and readily soluble in alcohol and ether. This body has been proved
to occur naturally in Coca leaves from various sources,
being present in some specimens as high as 0.5 per cent.

Thus it will be seen there has been much discussion and
uncertainty upon the Coca products, particularly so as to
those of an oily nature, originally designated as hygrine
and the amorphous substances previously described under
various titles.

# Volatile Principles

It is the opinion of Hesse that hygrine is a product of decomposition of one of the Coca bases, and does not occur
in fresh Coca leaves; in support of which he asserted that
while dilute acid solutions of hygrine have a strongly
marked blue florescence which is characteristic, this reaction is not shown when fresh leaves are first operated
upon. But as this reaction develops gradually, he inferred
that hygrine was formed by the decomposition of amorphous cocaine, from the solution of which it could be
separated by ammonia and caustic soda as a colorless oil
having the odor of quinoline. In fact, he considered the
oil thus obtained a homologue of quinoline, possibly a
tri-methyl-quinoline.

Another observer, while experimenting with the alkaloids of Coca by means of their platinum salts, obtained
an oily base, exceedingly bitter and differing in odor and
solubility from that which had been described by Lossen,
but which was presumably identical with the amorphous
products, cocwir cine and cocainiodine, and Hesse concluded there might really be two oily bases in amorphous
cocaine, one found in the benzoyl compounds of the
broad leaf variety and one in the cinnamyl compounds

of the Novo Granatense variety, in both cases associated with cocamine and another base, which he named cocrylamine. Liebermann, on the other hand, considers hygrine a combination of two liquid oxygenated bases

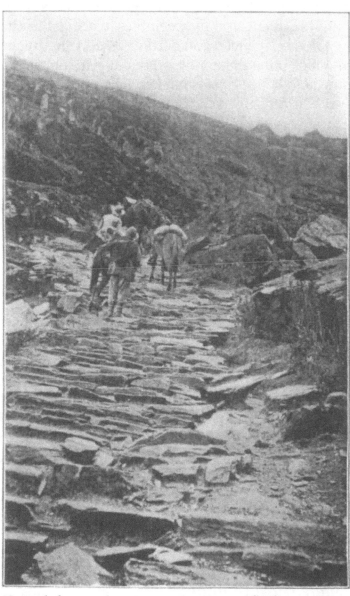

*Road from the Coca Region of Phara Peru*

which may be separated by fractional distillation. One—
$C_8H_{16}NO$, an isomeride of tropine, with a boiling point 193°
to 195°, the other, $C_{14}H_{24}N''_2O$, not distilling under ordinary
pressure without decomposition, while still other experimenters from distilling barium ecgonate obtained a volatile
oily liquid which strongly resembles hygrine. Merck has
shown this body yields, on decomposition, methylamine,
from which it has been inferred that it is identical with
tropine, and hence closely allied to atropine. With this fact in
view it was presumed the dilating property of cocaine upon
the pupil was due to hygrine, but this has been proved not
to be the case.

The assertion that hygrine is never present in Coca
leaves, but is merely a decomposition product in the manufacture of cocaine, lends an added interest to the research of
Dr. Rusby upon fresh Coca leaves made while he was at Bolivia. From repeated examinations he found a certain yield
of alkaloids, while specimens of the same leaves sent to the
United States yielded from treatment by the same process
less than half the percentage of alkaloid that he had obtained. This prompted him to search for the possible source
of error, and it was found that after all the cocaine was eliminated there was still a decided alkaloidal precipitate. From
this it was concluded that: "native Coca leaves contain
a body intimately associated with the cocaine and reacting
to the same test, which almost wholly disappears from them
in transit."

*The proportion of al-
kaloids contained in
Coca leaves is influ-
enced by the method of
the growth of the plant,
and the yield is depen-
dent upon the manner
of curing the leaves and
their preservation. The
percentage ranges from
a mere trace to about
one percent.*

This result indicates the
presence in Coca leaves of
some extremely volatile principle to which decided phys-

iological properties are attached, which may also be obtained from suitably preserved leaves. When a preparation made from recent leaves in Bolivia was submitted to Professor Remsen, of Johns Hopkins University, his assistant reported that he found a bitter principle, and an oil, which presumably differed in no way from that found at the time of the examinations made in Bolivia. This is comparable with similar findings of those who have experimented with Coca, whether the leaves were recent and examined on the spot, or the examination had been made thousands of miles distant upon well preserved leaves. In each instance similar volatile alkaloids have been obtained, which have commonly been pronounced "decomposition products," yet, as these are always found by careful observers, it indicates they are the natural associate bases of Coca.

The proportion of alkaloids contained in Coca leaves is influenced by the method of the growth of the plant, and the yield is dependent upon the manner of curing the leaves and their preservation. The percentage ranges from a mere trace to about one per cent. Bignon considers that well preserved leaves will yield fully as much as recent leaves, varying from nine to eleven grammes of the mixed alkaloids per kilogram, the latter being more than one per cent. Niemann obtained from his original process 0.25 per cent, of cocaine, while the present yield is more than double that. From a number of assays made during the last few years in the laboratory of an American manufacturer the following percentages of alkaloid were obtained: 0.53, 0.51, 0.63, 0.63, 0.57, 0.60, 0.66, 0.55, 0.70, 0.70, 0.65, 0.67, 0.54, 0.70, 0.32, 0.42, 0.52, 0.85, 0.48, 1.3, 0.78, 0.70, 0.40, 0.63. This will serve as an index of the quantity of total alkaloid commonly found in the average leaf of good quality as it reaches North America.

In determining the amount of alkaloids present in a given specimen of Coca, it is essential that the selected leaves be finely powdered, and mixed with a suitable menstruum that will not cause undue annoyance from gummy and resinous matters while setting free the essential constituents. These are washed out of the solution by an appropriate solvent, dried and weighed, or estimated by using some reagent the equivalent values of which have been determined by experiment. Various alkalies, as lime, soda or magnesia, have been suggested for admixture with the leaves for the purpose of liberating the alkaloids, which are transformed to soluble salts by acidulated water and washed out with strong alcohol. The details of the production of the Coca alkaloids commercially are kept as a trade secret, but the broad methods of manufacture are all similar, as several will illustrate.

Dr. Squibb has suggested the following process for the preparation of cocaine on a small scale:

> One hundred grammes of finely ground leaves are moistened with 100 c. c. of 7 per cent, solution of sodium carbonate, packed in a percolator, and sufficient kerosene added to make 700 c.c. of percolate. This is transferred to a separator, and 30 c.c. of 2 per cent, solution of hydrochloric acid added and shaken. After separation the watery solution is drawn off from below into a smaller separator, and this process is repeated three times, the alkaloid being in the smaller separator as an acid hydrochlorate. This is precipitated in ether with sodium carbonate, and evaporated at low heat with constant stirring and the product weighed.

Another process is to digest Coca leaves in a closed vessel at 70° C. for two hours with a very weak solution of caustic soda,and petroleum boiling between 200° to 250°. The mass is filtered, pressed while tepid, and the filtrate allowed to stand until the petroleum separates from the aqueous liquid. The former is then drawn off and neutralized with weak hydrochloric acid. The bulky precipitate of cocaine hydrochloride being recovered from the aqueous liquid by evaporation.

Gunn made a series of tests to determine what relation the methods of extraction had to the alkaloidal yield, and concluded that the modified method of Lyons obtained the most alkaloids. This is substantially as follows:

Shake 10 grammes of finely powdered leaves with 95 c.c. of petroleum benzin and add 5 c.c. of the following mixture: Absolute alcohol, 19 volumes; concentrated solution ammonia, 1 volume. Again shake for a few minutes, and set aside for twenty-four hours with occasional shaking. Decant rapidly 50 c.c. of the clear fluid, or, if it is not clear, filter it, washing the filter with benzin. Transfer to a separator containing 5 c.c. of water, to which has been added 6 to 8 drops of dilute sulphuric acid (1 to 5 by weight). Shake vigorously; when the fluids have separated draw the aqueous portion into a one ounce vial. Wash the contents of the separator with 2£ c.c. of acidulated water (1 drop of the dilute acid). Shake, draw off into the vial, and continue this two or three times, until a drop tested on a mirror with Mayer's reagent shows only faint turbidity. Add to the aqueous fluid 15 c.c. of benzin, shake, and when separation is complete, pour off the benzin. Add to the vial 15 c.c. of stronger ether, U. S. P., with sufficient ammonia to render the mixture decidedly alkaline. Shake, and when separation is complete, decant the ether carefully into a tared capsule. Wash the residue in the vial with two or three successive portions of fresh ether until the aqueous fluid is free from alkaloid, as shown by the test. Evaporate the ether over a water bath. Dry the alkaloid to constant weight, weigh, multiply the result expressed in decigrammes by two, which will present the percentage of crude cocaine.

Instead of extracting the alkaloid from the acid aqueous solution a simple method adapted to use in the field may be followed, in which the alkaloid is estimated by titration with Mayer's reagent. An acid solution representing 5 grammes of the leaves should be made up to a volume of 15 c.c, and the reagent added as long as it continues to precipitate in the clear filtrate. In this way, with half strength solution, 3.5 c.c. reagent represents 0.2 per cent, of alkaloid.

# Test for Cocaine

Mayer's reagent, or the decinormal mercuric potassium iodide of the U. S. P., is prepared as follows: Mercuric chloride, 13.546 grammes, dissolved in 600 c.c. of water; potassium iodide, 49.8 grammes, dissolved in 190 c.c. of water; mix the two solutions and add sufficient water to make the whole measure, at 59° F., exactly 1000 c.c.

When Mayer's reagent is added drop by drop to an acid solution containing cocaine (1:200 to 1:600) there is at first produced a heavy white precipitate, which collects at once into curdy masses; a drop of solution should be examined on a mirror, and should not show more than slight turbidity when determining the final traces. Dr. Lyons suggests that after adding a certain quantity of the reagent it will be found that the filtered fluid which still gives a heavy precipitate with Mayer's reagent produces a precipitate also in a fresh solution of cocaine. It is thus evident that the precipitation is complete only when an excess of reagent is present in the fluid; and it is found advisable to correct the reading from the burette by substracting for each c.c. of fluid present at the end of the titration 0.085 c.c. (if the half strength reagent is used); the remainder multiplied by ten will give the quantity of alkaloid indicated in milligrammes.   The best method of following the process is to throw the fluid on a filter after each addition of reagent. Solutions of the alkaloid 1:400 appear to yield better results than solutions stronger or weaker than this.

With Mayer's reagent used in half strength the following values for the equivalent of the reagent are given:

| Strength of cocaine solution. | 1 c.c. of Mayer's reagent (half strength) precipitates of cocaine. |
|---|---|
| 1:200 | 0.0062 |
| 1:300 | 0.0066 |
| 1:400 | 0.0070 |
| 1:500 | 0.0074 |
| 1:600 | 0.0078 |

## Quantity of Mayer's Reagent ($N_{20}^1$) Necessary to Precipitate a Given Quantity of Cocaine.

| Quantity of Cocaine | Measure of Fluid Titrated | | | |
|---|---|---|---|---|
| | 5 c.c. | 10 c.c. | 15 c.c. | 20 c.c. |
| .010 | 1.6 | | | |
| .020 | 2.7 | 3.1 | | |
| .030 | | 4.9 | 4.6 | |
| .040 | | 5.3 | 5.7 | 6.2 |
| .050 | | 6.4 | 6.8 | 7.3 |
| .060 | | | 7.9 | 8.4 |
| .070 | | | 9.0 | 9.5 |
| .080 | | | | 10.6 |
| .090 | | | | 11.7 |
| .100 | | | | 12.8 |
| | | | | |

One c.c. of Mayer's reagent will precipitate about 7.5 milligrammes of the mixed alkaloids from solutions in which alcohol is not present. As a rule the quantity of alkaloidal precipitate by this reagent is greater than the quantity of cocaine that can be extracted by washing out the alkaline solution with ether, so that in exact examinations a recourse to weighing is considered advisable. The dried precipitate weighed and multiplied by 0.406 will give about the amount of alkaloid present. Results higher or lower than those indicated are beyond the limits of the experiment and would call for repetition.

The principal tests employed to determine the purity of cocaine hydrochloride are the permanganate of potash and Maclagan's ammonia test. When one drop of a one

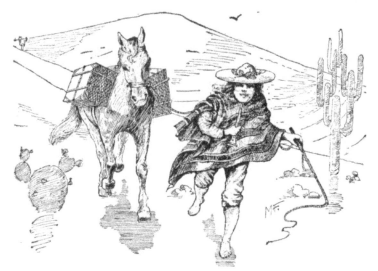

### *Indian Runner of the Andes*

per cent, solution of permanganate of potash is added to 5 c.c. of a two per cent, solution of hydrochloride of cocaine mixed with three drops of dilute sulphuric acid, it occasions a pink tint which should not entirely disappear within half an hour. When added to a stronger solution it occasions a precipitate of rhombic plates, which decompose on heating. If cinnamyl-cocaine be present the odor of bitter almonds is given off with the decomposition.

The Maclagan test is based upon the supposition that the amorphous alkaloids of Coca when set free by ammonia are separated as oily drops and so form a milky solution. It is employed by adding one or two drops of ammonia to a solution of cocaine, which is then vigorously stirred with a glass rod. If the salt is pure a formation of crystals will be deposited upon the rod and upon the side of the vessel within five minutes, while the solution will remain clear. If isatro-pyl-cocaine be present crystallization will not take place and the solution will become milky.

Considerable stress has been laid upon the value of this test for determining the purity of cocaine salts. Dr. Guenther asserts that a perfectly pure cocaine will not show the Maclagan reaction, while if a small quantity of a new base which he described as cocathylin, with a melting point of 110° C, be present, the test will be pronounced. In endeavoring to show that this was an error, one of the largest manufacturers of cocaine in Germany worked up four thousand kilos of Coca leaves, and though they failed to find the new base which had been mentioned, they also proved that a pure cocaine will respond positively to the Maclagan test. In support of this Paul and Cownley have expressed the opinion that any cocaine which does not satisfy this test should not be regarded as sufficiently pure for pharmaceutical purposes, views which are also maintained by E. Merck."

Of the various reagents that have been found delicate in testing for cocaine Mayer's reagent will detect one part in one hundred thousand, while a solution of iodine in iodide of potash will determine one part in four hundred thousand, with a very faint yellow precipitate.

# Assay of Crude Cocaine

It has been shown by Gerrard that mydriatic alkaloids have a peculiar action with mercuric chloride, from the aqueous solution of which they precipitate mercuric oxide, the other natural alkaloids giving no precipitate at all, or at least not separating mercuric oxide. The late Professor Fliickiger, verifying this action on cocaine, found the test recorded a very abundant purely white precipitate, which very speedily turned red, as in the case of the other mydriatic alkaloids.

It has been found, on treating cocaine or one of its salts in the solid state with fuming nitric acid, sp. gr. 1.4, evaporating to dryness and treating with one or two drops of strong alcoholic solution of potash, there is given off on stirring this with a glass rod a distinct odor suggestive of peppermint.   This odor test has been pronounced very delicate and is distinctive for cocaine, no other alkaloid having been found to yield a similar reaction.

There are several cocaine manufacturers in Peru. A few years ago there were five in Huanuco, one in the District of Mozon, one in Pozuso, two at Lima, one at Callao, at least two of which are run on an extensive scale. In 1894 the amount of the crude product manufactured in Peru and sent abroad for purification was four thousand seven hundred and sixteen kilos. A personal communication from Peru, dated January 15, 1900, states that the local manufacturers of cocaine are increasing their facilities and claim that they work with a better method than is followed elsewhere.

In 1890 Dr. Squibb called attention to the fact that crude cocaine was made so efficiently in Peru that it seemed highly probable that the importation of Coca leaves to this market was nearly at an end. This crude cocaine has a characteristic nicotine odor; it comes in a granular powder or in fragments of press cake, generally of a dull creamy white color, but rarely quite uniform throughout, the color ranging from dirty brownish white to very nearly white. Some of the fragments are horny, compact and hard, while others are softer and more porous.

## How to Determine the Amount of Cocaine Present in the Crude Product

A small quantity being taken from a large number of lumps in the parcels, selected on account of their difference in appearance, the determination of moisture in the samples so selected is found by fusion at 91° C. The solubility of the samples in ether at a specific gravity .725 at 15.6° C, is then tested. The insoluble residue is thoroughly washed with ether, dried and weighed. The alkaloid dissolved by the ether is converted into oxalate, and the oxalate shaken out by water. The residue which is soluble in ether is then determined by evaporation of the ethereal solution. The aqueous solution of cocaine oxalate is rendered faintly alkaline by soda; the freed alkaloid shaken out with ether, and after spontaneous evaporation of the ether and complete drying of the crystals produced, the pure alkaloid is estimated. The usual yield of pure crystallizable alkaloid from this crude product varies from fifty to seventy-five per cent.

Crude cocaine when united with acids assumes an intense green color, due to the presence of benzoyl-ecgonine, while its characteristic chemical reaction is its property of splitting into benzoic acid and methyl alcohol.

Cocaine combines readily with acids to form salts, which are readily soluble in water and alcohol, though insoluble in ether. These salts, owing to their more ready solubility, have a more marked anaesthetic action on mucous surfaces than the pure alkaloid. There has been prepared benzoate, borate, citrate, hydrobromate, hydrochlorate, nitrate, oleate, oxalate, salicylate, sulphate, tartrate, etc.

According to the U. S. Pharmacopoeia the following are the characteristics of cocaine hydrochlorate, the salt commonly employed:

"Colorless, transparent crystals, or a white crystalline powder, without odor, of a saline, slightly bitter taste, and producing upon the tongue a tingling sensation, followed by numbness of some minutes' duration. Permanent in the air. Soluble at 15° C. (59° F.) in 0.48 part of water and in 3.5 parts of alcohol; very soluble in boiling water and in boiling alcohol; also soluble in 2,800 parts of ether or in 17 parts of chloroform. On heating a small quantity of the powdered salt for twenty minutes at a temperature of 100° C. (212° F.), it should not suffer any material loss (absence of water of crystallization). The prolonged application of heat to the salt or to its solution induces decomposition. At 193° C. (379.4° F.) the salt melts with partial sublimation, forming a light brownish yellow liquid. When ignited it is consumed without leaving a residue. The salt is neutral to litmus paper."

In reviewing the research of many workers it may be seen how each has closely approached, often with a mere hint or suggestion, results which later have been verified and described more in detail. Through this repetition many new facts have been made positive to us. Assertions have been strengthened or have been cast aside, and while the result has been to render a cocaine of purer quality, it has at the same time emphasized the immensity of our ignorance concerning the subtleties of alkaloidal formation.

*Cocaine combines readily with acids to form salts, which are readily soluble in water and alcohol, though insoluble in ether.*

More than all, these researches must impress the fact that similar changes to those which are possible in the laboratory of the chemist are also at work in Nature's laboratory, and that the therapeutic influence and efficiency of Coca, as of any remedy taken into the body, must be markedly affected by the transmutations of the organism.

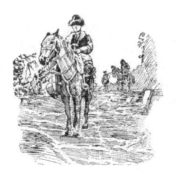

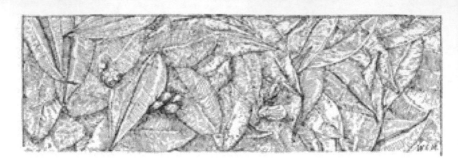

## Chapter 5

# Production of Alkaloids

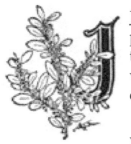 Just how alkaloids are produced in plants, while a subject full of interest to the chemist and physiologist, is one upon which our knowledge is not yet very exact.

The plants yielding alkaloids are widely distributed throughout the vegetable kingdom, belonging chiefly to the botanical division of dicotyledons. These substances are not found in the familiar *Graminiew* and *Labiatw,* and are rarely obtained in plants of the extensive order of composite, and thus far in only one family of the monocotyledons—the *Colchicece.*

## What Are Alkaloids

Alkaloids are nitrogenous carbon compounds, having basic properties, which are usually formed as the salts of organic acids. The greater number of them contain carbon, hydrogen, oxygen and nitrogen, though in a few cases oxygen is absent, and the resultant alkaloid is volatile, as nicotine, conine, sparteine, and some of the oily Coca bases.

*Chemically*, the vegetable alkaloids may be arranged in three groups, the first being derivatives of pyridine—as atropine and conine, the second derivatives of quinoline—as narcotine and cinchonine, the third those of the xanthin group—which are allied to urea, as caffeine. Nearly all the vegetable alkaloids belong to the first and second class, all of which contain nitrogen, and are probably formed by the action of ammonia, or amido compounds which are derived from ammonia, upon non-nitrogenous bodies.

Pyridine—$C_5H_5N$, may be regarded as a benzin—$C_0H_6$, in which one CH group has been replaced by one of nitrogen. The pyridine bases, metameric with aniline and its homologues, are contained in coal-tar, naphtha, tobacco smoke, and many organic substances. Konigs proposed confining the name alkaloid to plant derivatives of this origin. Quinoline—$C_9II_7N_3$, has the same relation to naphthalene—$C_{10}H_8$, that pyridine has to benzin; that is, it is derived by substituting one atom of nitrogen for one of the CH group in naphthalene.

# Vegtable Alkaloids

Originally an alkaloid was regarded merely as the active principle of the plant from which it was obtained, but as the number increased, and as allied substances were also found in animal tissues which were often spoken of as alkaloids, the general term has become confusional when applied to these bodies without regard to their derivation.With the advance in organic chemistry, which has enabled the building up of compounds from coal-tar products in the laboratory to intimately resemble the true plant bases, it is often important to distinguish between those alkaloids which are natural and those which are of artificial production. Yet this very fact has indicated the correlation of all matter, and the investigations of the chemist and physiologist have happily progressed together, each furthering the research of the other.

Aristotle attempted to trace an absolute connection between all living things, and though it would seem that one might immediately pronounce to which class an organism belongs, it is really not so simple.

The lower forms of one so nearly approach the lower forms of the other order that biologists have often found extreme difficulty in determining a classification that shall be generally accepted by naturalists.

The old illustration as showing the distinction between plants and animals, that the former absorb carbonic acid and give off oxygen, while animals do just the reverse, is only partially true, for while it is a fact that animals give off carbonic acid, plants cannot live in the absence of oxy-

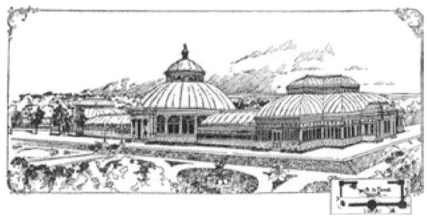

### *Conservatories of New York Botanical Garden at Bronx Park*

gen, which is essential to furthering the processes of their metabolism. As another illustration, it was shown that plants have not the power of voluntary motion possessed by animals, but this assertion was shown to be wrong by numerous examples among the lower forms, which are precisely the reverse. All individual cells must possess the power of motion, and some of the lower plant organisms actually move from place to place—indeed, locomotion is absolutely necessary to their existence. On the other hand, some lower animal structures are permanently fixed, so that the older comparisons are not definite. Similar chemical changes take place in the cell structure of plants and animals. All must have motion incidental to growth, together with the functions of sleep, nutrition and irritability, which latter property is manifest by certain plants to a remarkable degree under the influence of such nitrogenous foods as raw meat, milk or albumen.

As vegetable alkaloids are considered to be the excreta of plants, we cannot properly draw any conclusion concerning their probable formation without regarding the changes, which are brought about in the life of the organism producing them. As these processes are intimately allied to changes which are undergone under similar conditions in the animal being, a review of the subject may not be wholly uninteresting, while it will enable us to more fully appreciate the possible action of the products of the Coca leaf when we come to consider the application of that interesting plant more directly in the human economy.

All organic structure is built up through a constant breaking down and rearrangement of simple chemical elements. In the case of plants, the compounds of the elements, which have been admixed with the soil are carried in solution through the root to the most remote cells of the leaf. There these chemical bodies are converted into complex substances, which under suitable stimuli are built to form the tissues of the organism. These subtle changes take place only under the influence of that mighty alchemist, the sun.

It would seem that the Incas were not far wrong in regarding this great source of light and activity as at least the physical source of all power, for not only is

*All organic structure is built up through a constant breaking down and rearrangement of simple chemical elements.*

plant life dependent upon the action of the sun, but the animal being is in turn dependent upon plant structure. Those compounds which have been so mysteriously molded into vegetable organisms must be torn apart and dissolved in order to set free the elements of which animal structure is composed. Here these elements are rearranged to the necessities of a higher organization, where they may continue a still more complex existence. This constant interchange is carried on through plants and animals—through animals and plants—each organism converting and reconverting, from age to age, the various elements appropriate to its own requirements. In the performance of these functional processes, each cell of the tissues creates for itself, as well as for surrounding bodies, that combination of energy, which we call life. These changes are carried on without intermediary loss of matter—which we know is indestructible—regardless of the extent or method of the many conversions it may have undergone since creation, and shall continue to undergo until the end of time.

# Principal Elements

There are four principal elements of the sixty-seven or more known ones, which may be regarded as the very basis of life. These are carbon, hydrogen, oxygen and nitrogen, and all organic changes take place in accordance with the varying proportions that these elements unite with each other. Carbon we are apt to carelessly regard as that coke-like substance made familiar to us through its employment in electricity, without stopping to recall its important relation to all organic tissue. It enters into the building of other cells than electric, for it is found, without exception, in every tissue of organic life. It seems difficult to understand how so apparently inert a substance can become intimately incorporated with living structures. Carbon, which as a product of combustion is everywhere diffused as carbonic acid, is carried as a gas and in solution to the plant and is absorbed by the roots and stomata of the leaves. Here under sunshine it is deposited for immediate use or to form emergency food for the tissues, while the oxygen is set free to again enter into the performance of those multiple chemical processes included in growth and decay. So important is the influence of carbon in all organic structures that Pniiger has advanced the theory that carbon united with nitrogen as cyanogen constituted the radical which formed the very nucleus of creation—of that molten chaos from which all existence sprung.

*Nitrogen may be regarded, if not the source of all energy, certainly as the chemical creator of force, for it is absolutely necessary in all compounds from which power is to be derived.*

Nitrogen may be regarded, if not the source of all energy, certainly as the chemical creator of force, for it is absolutely necessary in all compounds from which power is to be derived. The changes due to oxygen are so much more spoken of that it would seem the importance of nitrogen is often disregarded. Though everywhere about us this element cannot, like oxygen, be readily forced into union, and plants cannot take in free nitrogen. But so essential is this subtle element to all organic energies through its formation of proteids and their decomposition, that it must be coaxed into suitable combinations by similar transmutations as those for the deposit of carbon—the activity of vegetable life under the stimulus of sunshine. Its combinations, however, are loose and maintained with difficulty, yet this very effort for constant freedom causes this to be the most important element of all chemical compounds in which it is associated. The property of nitrogen of escaping from union and liberating energy is made use of in the high explosives, and is also exhibited in the more subtle decom-

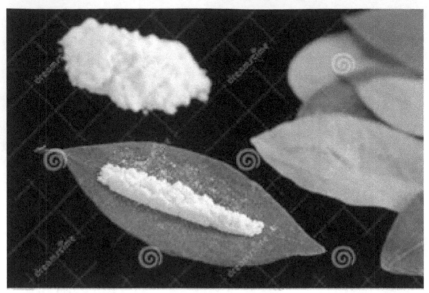

### *Cocaine Powder*

positions of decay, which owe their potency to the nitrogen contained in their ammonia.

Similar changes due to the influence of nitrogen are constantly going on in the processes of metabolism in all organic tissue. We have an instance of this when the carbohydrates of plants are converted into proteid structures, which, decomposing, again set free their nitrogen as excreta in the form of alkaloids. Again this property is shown in the human laboratory when the pent-up nitrogen in the Coca leaf is brought to bear upon the customary maize dietary of the Andean, and as a result the starchy elements are converted into the more complex molecule of the flesh-forming proteid.

With these four primary elements are mingled others, including sulphur, phosphorus, potassium, calcium, magnesium, iron, and the gaseous element chlorine, all of which may serve to nourish certain tissues of the organism to which they are carried in solution of various compounds. So while the several primary elements are essential to the structure of every organism, it is impossible for them to be utilized in the upbuilding of tissue until carried to the cell in fluid form. In the case of plant life, the elements are conveyed in such dilution of their salts that their presence is seemingly physically absent, while the fluids are apparently but simple water. This solution is taken up from the soil through the roots, yet the selection may not be only of such substances as are of positive nutritive value, but of other substances in solution, which may even be injurious.

Though the structural formation may be different, it is nevertheless true that all tissue is built up of cells—modified in form or function, and all organic life is but an aggregation of the cell which thus constitutes the unit of existence. The various changes of growth and decay are to be observed through these cells—whether of bone, of wood, of muscle or of leaf, and the comparative study under the microscope of these primary tissues emphasizes the assurance that all the world is akin. The cell is in fact the beginning of life for both animals and plants, and the organism is but an aggregation or community of these primitive parts. So alike indeed are the embryonic cells, as Karl von Baer, in 1828, pointed out, that the various species cannot be determined from any differences discernible, even by the aid of the most powerful microscope. From this it would seem but an easy gradation to infer the doctrine of evolution. All change in life is akin to the change within these little cells due to the taking in and excretion of matter in which carbonic acid plays a most important part.

In the Coca leaf, as indeed in all plants, the cell wall is made up of cellulose, a carbohydrate substance allied to starch, with the formula $xC_6H_{10}O_5$. The material for the building of this substance, it is presumed, is secreted by the cell contents or by a conversion of protoplasm under the influence of nitrogen. This product is deposited particle by particle inside of the wall already formed. Accompanying this growth there may occur certain changes in the physical

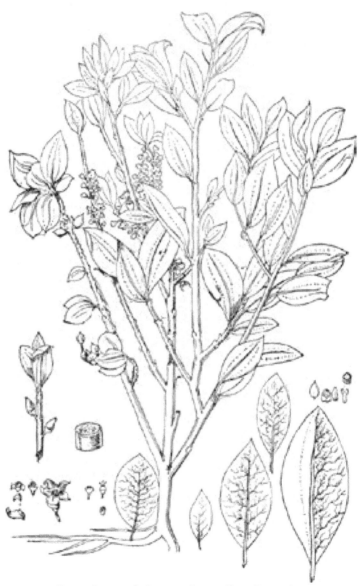

*Species of Coca Sent by Jussieu*

properties of the cell as the wall takes in new substances, such as silica and various salts, or as there is an elaboration and deposit of gum, pectose and lignin. Each living cell contains a viscid fluid, of extremely complex chemical composition—the protoplasm—a layer of which is in contact with the cell wall and connected by bridles with a central mass in which the nucleus containing the nucleolus is embedded. The protoplasm does not fill the whole cavity of the cell, but there is a large space filled with the watery sap.

The sap carries in solution certain sugars, together with glycogen and two varieties of glucose, and such organic acids and coloring matters as may already have been elaborated. Where metabolism is active, certain crystallizable nitrogenous bodies, as asparagin, leucin and tyrosin, with salts of potassium and sodium, are found, while in the vacuole there may be starch grains and some crystals of calcium oxalate. The protoplasm is chemically made up of proteids, of which two groups may be distinguished in plants. The first embracing the plastin, such as forms the frame work of the cell, and the second the peptones of the seeds, and the globulins found in the buds and in young shoots. These proteids all consist of carbon, hydrogen, nitrogen, oxygen, and sulphur, while plastin also contains phosphorus. In active growing cells the proteids are present in a quantity, which gradually diminishes as the cell becomes older, leaving the plastin as the organized proteid wall of the cell, while the globulins and peptones remain unorganized. The whole constructive metabolism of the plant is toward the manufacture of this protoplasm, the chemical decomposition and conversion of which liberates the energy, which continues cell life.

# Influence of Chlorophyl

In certain cells of the plant associated with the protoplasm, and presumably of a similar chemical composition, are

little corpuscles, which contain the chlorophyl constituting
the green coloring matter of plants, a substance which from
its chemical construction and physiological function may
have some important influence on the alkaloid formation
in the Coca leaf. In these bodies the chlorophyl is held in an
oily medium, which exudes in viscid drops when the granules are treated with dilute acids or steam. Although no
iron has been found in these bodies by analysis, it is known
that chlorophyl cannot be developed without the presence
of iron in the soil. Gautier, from an alcoholic extract, calculated the formula $C_{19}H_{22}N_2O_3$, and called attention to the
similarity between this and that of bilirubin, $C_{16}H_{18}N_2O_3$—
the primary pigment forming the golden red color of the
human bile, which possibly may be allied to the red corpuscles of the blood.

Chlorophyl, while commonly only formed under appropriate conditions of light and heat, may in some cases
be produced in complete darkness, in a suitable temperature. Thus if a seed be made to germinate in the dark, the
seedling will be not green, but pale yellow, and the plant
is anomic, or is termed etiolated, though corpuscles are
present, which, under appropriate conditions, will give rise
to chlorophyl.

It has been found that etiolated plants become green
more readily in diffused light than in bright sunshine. The
process of chlorophyl formation neither commences directly
when an etiolated plant is exposed to light, nor ceases entirely when a green plant is placed in darkness, but the action
continues through what has been termed photo-chemical
induction. From experiments to determine the relative efficacy of different rays of the spectrum it has been found that
in light of low intensity seedlings turn green more rapidly
under yellow rays, next under green, then under red, and
less rapidly under blue. In intense light the green formation
is quicker under blue than under yellow, while under the
latter condition decomposition is more rapid.

The function of chlorophyl is to break up carbonic acid, releasing oxygen, and converting the carbon into storage food for the tissues, the first visible stage of which constructive metabolism is the formation of starch. The activity of this property may be regarded as extremely powerful when it is considered that in order to reduce carbonic acid artificially it requires the extraordinary temperature of 1300° C. (2372° F.). In the leaf this action takes place under the influence of appropriate light and heat from the sun in the ordinary temperature of 10°-30° C. (50°-86°F.). Plants, which do not contain chlorophyl—as fungi—obtain their supply of carbon through more complex compounds in union with hydrogen.

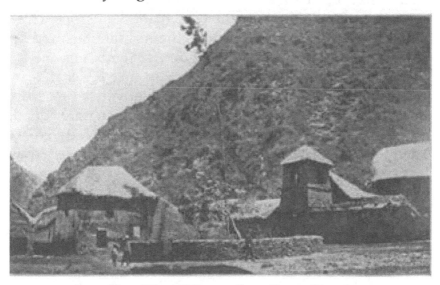

### Sandia, Peru Near the Coca Region

Perhaps we are too apt to regard plants as chiefly cellulose—-carbohydrates, and water, without considering the importance of their nitrogenous elements, for though these latter substances may be present in relatively small proportion, they are as essential in the formation of plant tissue as in animal structures. The carbohydrates of plants include starch, sugars, gums, and inulin. The starch or an allied

substance, as has been shown, being elaborated by the
chlorophyl granules, or in those parts of the plant where
these bodies do not exist, by special corpuscles in the protoplasm, termed *amyloplasts,* which closely resemble the chlorophyl bodies. In the first instance the change is more simple and
under the influence of light, in the latter light is not directly
essential and the process is more complex, the starch formation
beginning with intermediate substances—as asparagin, or glucose, by conversion of the sugars in the cell sap.

Just as in the human organism, assimilation in plant
tissue cannot take place except through solution, so the
stored up starch is of no immediate service until it is rendered soluble. In other words, it must be prepared in a way
analogous to the digestion of food in animal tissues. This
is done by the action of certain ferments manufactured
by the protoplasm. These do not directly enter into the
upbuilding of tissue themselves, but induce the change in
the substance upon which they act. Chiefly by a process of
hydration, in which several molecules of water are added,
the insoluble bodies are rendered soluble, and are so carried in solution to various portions of the plant. Here they
are rearranged as insoluble starch, to serve as the common
storage tissue for sustenance. Thus it will be seen how very
similar are the processes of assimilation in plants and animals, a marked characteristic between both being that the
same elementary chemical substances are necessary in the
upbuilding of their tissues, and particularly that activity is
absent where assimilable nitrogen is not present.

# Organic Acids

Several organic acids occur in plant cells, either free or
combined, which are probably products of destructive
metabolism, either from the oxidation of carbohydrates or
from the decomposition of proteids. Liebig regarded the
highly oxidized acids—especially oxalic, as being the first

products of constructive metabolism, which, by gradual reduction, formed carbohydrates and fats, in support of which he referred to the fact that as fruits ripen they become less sour, which he interpreted to mean that the acid is converted into sugar. The probability, however, is that oxalic

*Oxalic acid is very commonly found in the leaf cells combined with potassium or calcium.*

acid is the product of destructive metabolism, and is the final stage of excretion from which alkaloids are produced, while it is significant, when considering the Coca products, that acids may by decomposition be formed from proteid or may by oxidation be converted into other acids.

Oxalic acid is very commonly found in the leaf cells combined with potassium or calcium. It is present in the cells of the Coca leaf as little crystalline cubes or prisms. Malic acid, citric acid, and tartaric acid are familiar as the products of various fruits. Tannic acid is chiefly found as the astringent property of various barks. Often a variety of this acid is characteristic of the plant and associated with its alkaloid. This is the case with the tannic acid described by Niemann in his separation of cocaine, which is intimately related to the alkaloids of the Coca leaf, just as quinine is combined with quinic acid and morphine with meconic acid. It has been suggested that the yield of alkaloid from the Coca leaf is greater in the presence of a large proportion of tannic acid.

# Tannin

Tannin is formed in the destructive metabolism of the protoplasm, as a glucoside product intermediate between the carbohydrate and the purely aromatic bodies, such as benzoic and cinnamic acids, which are formed from the oxidative decomposition of the glucosides. In addition to these are found fatty oils, associated with the substances of the cell, and essential oils, to which the fragrance of the flower or plant is due, and which are secreted in special walled cells. The resins are found as crude resins, balsams—a mixture of resin and ethereal oil with an aromatic acid, and gum resins—a mixture of gum, resin and ethereal oil. The ethereal oils include a great number of substances with varying chemical composition, having no apparent constructive use to the tissues, but, like the alkaloids, regarded merely as waste. Some of these products serve by their unpleasant properties to repel animals and insects, while others serve to attract insects and thus contribute to the fertilization of the flower, so all these bodies may be of some relative use.

The proteids of the plant are supposed to be produced from some non-nitrogenous substance—possibly formic aldehyde—by a combination formed from the absorbed nitrates, sulphates and phosphates, in union with one of the organic acids, particularly oxalic. The change being from the less complex compound to a highly nitrogenous organic substance, termed an amide, which, with the non-nitrogenous substance and sulphur, unite to form the proteid. The amides are crystallizable nitrogenous substances, built up synthetically, or formed by the breaking down of certain compounds. They are similar to some of the final decomposition products found in the animal body. Belonging to this group of bodies is xanthin, which Kossel supposed to be directly derived from nuclein, from the nucleus of the plant cell. But in whatever manner the amides are formed, it is believed they are ultimately used in the construction of proteid, and although this substance is produced in all parts of the plant, it is found more abundant in the cells containing chlorophyl. Proteids are found to gradually increase from the roots toward the leaves, where they are most abundant. This would seem to indicate that the leaf is the especial organ in which proteid formation takes place, and it is in this portion of the Coca plant that the excreted alkaloids are found most abundantly.

According to Schiitzenberger, the proteid structures are composed of ureids, derivatives of carbamide, and Grimaux considers they are broken by hydrolysis into carbonic acid, ammoniac and amidic acids, thus placing them in near relation with uric acid, which also gives by hydrolysis, carbonic acid, ammoniac acid and glycocol. In animal tissues the last product of excrementition is carbamide—or uric acid, while the compounds from which proteids are formed in plants have been shown to be amides. It has been shown in the laboratory that the chemical products from the breaking down of proteids are also amides, with which carbonic acid and oxalic acid are nearly always formed. The presence of hippuric acid in the urine of herbivorous animals, the indol and the skatol found in the products of pancreatic digestion (Salkowski), together with the tyrosin nearly always present in the animal body, has led to the supposition that aromatic groups may also be constituents of the proteid molecule.

# Nitrogen.

All of this is of the greatest interest in the study of alkaloid production in connection with the fact, which has been proved, that when a plant does not receive nitrogen from outside it will not part with the amount of that element previously contained—in other words, the nitrogenous excreta will not be thrown off. Boussingault thought the higher plants flourished best when supplied with nitrogen in the form of nitrates, though Lehmann has found that many plants flourish better when supplied with ammonia salts than when supplied with nitrates, and this has been well marked in the case of the tobacco plant.

Nitric acid may be absorbed by a plant in the form of any of its salts, which can diffuse into the tissues, the most common bases being soda, potash, lime, magnesia and ammonia. The formation of this acid, attendant upon the electric conditions of the atmosphere, may be one source of increase of vigor to the native soil of the Coca plant, where the entire region of the montana is so subject to frequent electrical storms. Then Coca flourishes best in soils rich in humus, and various observers have remarked that nitrogen is best fixed in such a soil. An interesting point in connection with which is that the ammonia supplied to the soil by decomposition of nitrogenous substances is converted into nitrous, and this into nitric acid, by a process termed

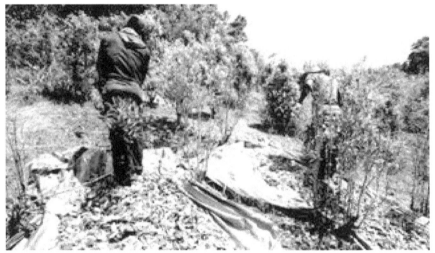

*Coca Harvesting*

nitrification, occasioned by the presence of certain bacteria in the soil to which this property is attributed. Proof of this was determined by chloroforming a section of nitrifying earth and finding that the process on that area ceased. The absorption of nitrogen by the Coca plant and the development of proteids is closely associated with the nitrogenous excreta from the plant, and the consequent production of alkaloids which we are attempting to trace.

The nitrogen of the soil, however induced, is transferred by oxidation into what has been termed the reduced nitrogen of amides, which, in combination with carbohydrates, under appropriate conditions forms proteids, in which oxalic acid is an indirect product. Several observers consider the leaves as active in this process, because the nitrogenous compounds are found to accumulate in the leaf until their full development, when they decrease. This is illustrated by the fact that in autumn, when new proteids are not necessary to matured leaves, it accumulates in the protoplasm, from which it is transferred to the stem, to be stored up as a food for the following season's growth.

It has been found that the nitrates, passing from the roots as calcium nitrate, are changed in the leaves by the chloropliyl in the presence of light with the production of calcium oxalate, while nitric acid is set free, and conversely, In darkness the nitrates are permitted to accumulate. This change is influenced by the presence of oxalic acid, which, even in small quantities, is capable of decomposing the most dilute solutions of calcium nitrate. The free nitric acid in combination with a carbohydrate forms the protein molecule, while setting free carbonic acid and water.

Cellulose, which we have seen is formed from protoplasm, is dependent upon the appropriate conversion of the nitrogenous proteid. When this formation is active, large amounts of carbohydrates are required to form anew the protein molecule of the protoplasm, and the nitrogenous element is utilized. When there is an insufficiency of carbohydrate material the relative amount of nitrogen increases because the conditions are not favorable for its utilization in the production of proteids, and this excess of nitrogen is converted into amides, which are stored up. When the carbohydrate supply to the plant is scanty in amount this reserve store of amides is consumed, just the same as the reserve fat would be consumed in the animal structure under similar conditions.

The relation between the normal use of nitrogen in plants is analogous to its influence in animal structure, while the final products in both cases are similar, the distinction being chiefly one in the method of chemical conversion and excretion due to the difference in organic function. Thus, although urea and uric acid are not formed in plants, the final products of both animals and plants are closely allied. We see this especially in the alkaloids caffeine and theobromine, which are almost identical with uric acid, so much so that Haig considers that a dose of caffeine is equivalent to introducing into the system an equal amount of uric acid.

There are numerous examples, not only in medicinal substances, but in the more familiar vegetables and fruits, which illustrate the possibilities of change due to cultivation. The Siberian rhododendron varies its properties from stimulant to a narcotic or cathartic, in accordance with its location of growth. Aconite, assafoetida, cinchona, digitalis, opium and rhubarb are all examples which show the influence of soil and cultivation.

Indeed similar effects are to be seen everywhere about us, certain characteristics being prominently brought forth by stimulating different parts of the organism, so that ultimately distinct varieties are constituted. The poisonous Persian almond has thus become the luscious peach. The starchy qualities of the potato are concentrated in its increased tuber, and certain poisonous mushrooms have become edible. The quality of the flour from wheat is influenced by locality and cultivation. The tomato, cabbage, celery, asparagus, are all familiar examples which emphasize the possibility of shaping nature's wild luxuriance to man's cultured necessity.

The chemical elements which are taken up by a plant vary considerably with the conditions of environment, and the influence of light in freeing acid in the leaf has been indicated. These conditions necessarily modify the constituents of the plant. When metabolism is effected certain changes take place in the tissues, with the formation of substances which may be undesirable to the plant, yet may

be medicinally serviceable. Such a change occurs in the
sprouts of potatoes stored in the dark, when the poisonous
base *solania* is formed, which under normal conditions of
growth is not present in the plant. A familiar example of
change due to environment is exhibited in the grape, which
may contain a varying proportion of acid, sugar and salts
in accordance with the soil, climate and conditions of its
cultivation, nor are these variations merely slight, for they
are sufficient to generate in the wine made from the fruit
entirely different tastes and properties.

In view of these facts, it seems creditable to suppose
that by suitable processes of cultivation the output of alkaloids may be influenced in plants, and such experiments
have already been extensively carried out in connection
with the production of quinine. When attention was directed to the scientific cultivation of cinchona in the East, it
was remarked that when manured with highly nitrogenous
compounds the yield of alkaloid was greatly increased.
This is paralleled by the fact that when an animal consumes a large quantity of nitrogenous food the output of
urea and uric acid is greater.

Alkaloids are regarded as waste products because they
cannot enter into the constructive metabolism of the plant,
though they are not directly excreted, but are stored away
where they will not enter the circulation, and may be soon
shed, as in the leaf or bark. Though, as indicating their possible utility, it has been shown experimentally that plants
are capable of taking up nitrogenous compounds, such as
urea, uric acid, leucin, tyrosin, or glycocol, when supplied
to their roots. In some recent experiments carried out at
the botanical laboratory of Columbia University, I found
that plant metabolism was materially hastened under the
stimulus of cocaine.

# Physical Influrences

The influence of light in the formation of alkaloids has already been shown. Tropical plants which produce these substances in abundance in their native state often yield but small quantities when grown in hot houses, indicating that a too intense light is unfavorable, probably in stimulating a too rapid action of the chlorophyl, together with a decomposition of the organic acid. Some years ago the botanist, Dr. Louis Errera, of Brussels, found that the young leaves of certain plants yielded more abundant alkaloid than those that were mature. Following this suggestion, Dr. Greshoff is said to have found that young Coca leaves yield nearly double the amount of alkaloid over that contained in old leaves gathered at the same time. In tea plantations the youngest leaves are gathered, but it has always been customary to collect the mature leaves of the Coca plant,

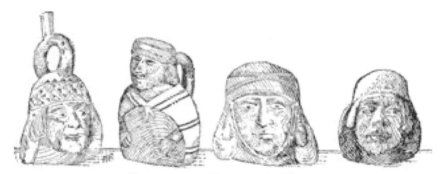

*Peruvian Protrait Vases*

and these have usually been found to yield the greatest amount of alkaloid. The probability is that the amount of alkaloid present in the Coca leaf is not so much influenced by maturity as it is by the period of its gathering.

As regards the temperature at which growth progresses most favorably, Martins has compared each plant to a thermometer, the zero point of which is the minimum temperature at which its life is possible. Thus, the Coca shrub in its native state will support a range from 18° C. (64.4° F.) to 30° C. (86° F.), an influence of temperature which is governed by the proportion of water contained in the plant. It has been found, from experiments of cultivation, that Coca will flourish in a temperature considerably higher than that which was originally supposed bearable, though the alkaloidai yield is less than that grown more temperately. The life process of any plant, however, may be exalted as the temperature rises above its zero point, though only continuing to rise until a certain height is reached, at which it ceases entirely. In the cold, plants may undergo a similar hibernation as do certain animals when metabolism is lessened, though long-continued cold is fatal, and frost is always so absolutely to Coca. The influence of temperature on metabolism tends to alter the relations between the volume of carbonic acid given off and the amount of oxygen absorbed. Under a mean temperature these relations are equal, while in a lower temperature more oxygen is absorbed in proportion to the carbonic acid given off, and oxygen exhalation ceases entirely below a certain degree.

A relatively large proportion of water in a plant determines its susceptibility to climatic conditions. Thus freezing not only breaks the delicate parenchymatous tissues, but alters the chemical constitution of the cells, while too high a temperature may prove destructive through a coagulation of the albumen. The appearance of plants killed by high or low temperature being similar. Roots are stimulated to curve to their source of moisture, and their power for absorption is more active in a high than in a low temperature, but as absorption is influenced by the transpiration of the plant, it is less active in a moist atmosphere, unless the metabolic processes of the plant occasions a higher temperature than the surrounding air. Such activity would be increased by the heat of the soil about the roots, and is probably manifest in the Coca plant through the peculiar soil of the montana.

The elevation at which a plant grows has an influence upon the absorption by the leaf. Thus it has been observed that while a slight increase in the carbonic acid gas contained in the air is favorable to growth, a considerable increase is prejudicial, while an increase or diminution of atmospheric pressure materially influences plant life. In some tropical countries Coca will grow at the level of the sea, provided there is an equable temperature and requisite humidity. Although in Peru Coca flourishes side by side with the best coffee, it will not thrive at the elevations where the coffee plant is commonly grown in either the East or West Indies. In Java, where experiments have been made in cultivating Coca, it has been stated that there is no perceptible difference in the alkaloidal yield due to the influence of elevation, while in the best cocals of Peru it is considered that the higher the altitude at which Coca can be grown the greater will be the alkaloidal yield. This is possibly effected by similar influences to that governing the aromatic properties developed in the coffee bean, which have been found more abundant when coffee is grown at an elevation, yet without danger of frost. This may be attributed to slower growth and a consequent deposit of nitrogenous principles instead of their being all consumed through a rapid metabolism.

It is therefore evident that as these several physical conditions have a marked bearing upon the life history of all plants, the more limited the range for any of these processes in any particular plant, the more it will be influenced. Thus in an altitude too high, the leaf of the Coca plant is smaller and only one harvest is possible within the year, while in the lower regions where the temperature exceeds 20° C. (68° F.) vegetation may be exuberant, but the quality of leaf is impaired. The electrical conditions of the atmosphere, it has been shown, have an important bearing upon the development of Coca, through the influence of the gases set free in the atmosphere and the possible slight increase of nitric acid carried to the soil.

It was thought by Martius that the mosses and lichens which are found upon the Coca shrubs were detrimental to the plant through favoring too great humidity. In the light of our knowledge on the development of alkaloids, however, it has seemed to me that here is an opportunity for very extended experimentation, as may be inferred from a reference to the alkaloidal production of cinchona. At first efforts were made to free the cinchona trees from the lichens and mosses which naturally formed upon them; but it was discovered accidentally that those portions of the trees which Nature had covered in this manner yielded an increased amount of alkaloid. When cinchona plantations were started in Java, experiments made upon the result of this discovery prompted a systematic covering of the trunks of the trees artificially with moss, which was bound about them to the height from which the bark would be stripped. At first very great pains was taken to collect just an appropriate kind of moss, which it was supposed from its association with the tree in its native home would be essential, but later experiments proved that any form of covering which protected the bark from light increased this alkaloidal yield. So that today this process, which is known as "mossing," is one of the most important in the cultivation and development of cinchona.

# Cultivation of Alkaloids

The chief interest of Coca to the commercial world has centered upon its possibilities in the production of the one alkaloid, cocaine, instead of a more general economic use of the leaf. Because of this, much confusion of terms has resulted, for chemists have designated the amount of alkaloids obtained from the leaf as cocaine, although they have qualified their statement by saying that a portion of this is uncrystallizable. Numerous experiments have been conducted to determine the relative yield of cocaine from

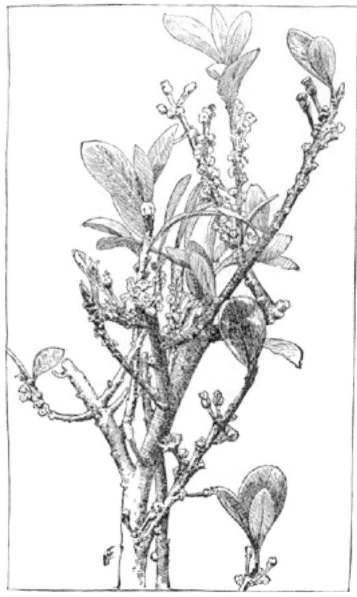

*Bolivian Coca*

the different varieties of Coca, and when uncrystallizable alkaloids have been found the leaf has been condemned for chemical uses. It will thus be appreciated how a great amount of error has been generated and continued. The Bolivian or Huanuco variety has been found to yield the largest percentage of crystallizable alkaloid, while the Peruvian or Truxillo variety, though yielding nearly as much total alkaloid, affords a less percentage that is crystallizable, the Bolivian Coca being set apart for the use of the chemists to the exclusion of the Peruvian variety, which is richest in aromatic principles and best suited for medicinal purposes. As a matter of fact, the Peruvian Coca is the plant sought for by the native users.

There is not only a difference in the yield of alkaloid from different varieties of Coca, but also a difference in the yield from plants of one variety from the same cocal, and it would seem possible by selection and propagation of the better plants to obtain a high percentage of alkaloid. At present there is no effort in the native home of Coca toward the production of alkaloid in the leaf through any artificial means. Regarding the quality of alkaloid that has been found in the different plants, the Peruvian variety has been found to contain equal proportions of crystallizable and uncrystallizable alkaloid, while the Bolivian variety contains alkaloids the greater amount of which are crystallizable cocaine. Plants, which are grown in conservatory, even with the greatest care, yield but a small percentage of alkaloid, of which, however, the uncrystallizable alkaloid seems more constant while the relative amount of cocaine is diminished. In leaves grown at Kew .44 per cent, of alkaloid was obtained, of which .1 per cent, was crystallizable. From experiments of Mr. G. Peppe, of Renchi, Bengal, upon leaves obtained from plants imported from Paris, it was found that leaves dried in the sun yielded .53 per cent, of alkaloid, of which .23 per cent, was uncrystallizable. The same leaves dried in the shade on cloth for twenty hours, then rolled by hand, after the manner in which Chinese tea is treated, then cured for two and a half hours and dried over a charcoal fire and packed in close tins, yielded .58 per cent, of alkaloid, of which .17 per cent, was uncrystallizable.

It is probable that each variety of Coca has a particular range of altitude at which it may be best cultivated. The Bolivian variety is grown at a higher altitude than Peruvian Coca, while the Novo Granatense variety has even been found to thrive at the level of the sea. Among Coca, as among the *cinchona,* certain varieties yield a large proportion of total alkaloids, of which only a small amount is crystallizable. The *Cinchona succirubra* yields a large amount of mixed alkaloids, but a small amount of quinine, while *Cinchona Calisaya* yields a smaller amount of mixed alkaloids and a large amount of crystallizable quinine. A few authors who have referred to the alkaloidal yield of Coca leaves have casually remarked that the plants grown in the shade produce an increased amount above those grown in the sun, which would appear to be paralleled by the formation of chlorophyl and the production of proteids, both of which have so important a bearing upon the metabolism of the plant and the final nitrogenous excretion.

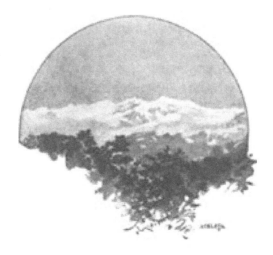

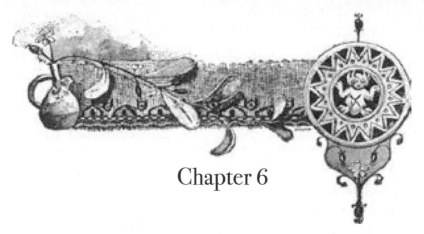

## Chapter 6

# Coca & Muscular Energy

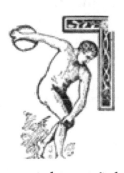 HERE has been no period since the command was given Adam in the Garden of Eden, when physical exertion was not essential to existence. The ancient philosophers instilled the doctrine that a sound mind is only possible in a sound body, and so Homer pictured the dejection of Achilles as eating his own heart in idleness because he might not fight. Idleness has ever been so recognized as a common precursor of discontent and melancholia, that when the children of Israel murmured against Pharaoh their tasks were wisely doubled to prevent retrospection. Occupation is not only essential to prosperity, but is morally and physically conducive to health and longevity and a rest is best attained not by total cessation, but by a change of employment. I believe it was Hammond who advised a wealthy neurasthenic to collect used corks, with the result that the patient became so interested in this unique occupation that his brooding was soon forgotten, while he became an expert in old stoppers.

With a popular regard for the benefits of appropriate exercise, the matter of athletics has been greatly overdone, and has often resulted in injury instead of the anticipated good. The early Greeks, who elaborated every form of gymnastics, only undertook the severe strain incidental to their games after a suitable preparatory period. They were encouraged to these performances—which were instituted in honor of the gods or deified heroes—through the idea that they were sacred, and in fulfillment of this the exercises always began with a sacrifice, and concluded in the same religious manner. In the period of Cassar, a victory in the Olympic games was considered such a triumph that honors were not only extended to the victor, but to his relatives and even to his place of birth. There was, however, no impromptu emulation permitted in these contests, but those who desired to compete were obliged to submit themselves for preparatory practice at least ten months before the exercises began.

## Althletics Overdone

"Wherever there is an incentive for supremacy, there is a possibility of overstrain, and Hippocrates cautioned the athletes against the possible error of immoderate exercise. Galen foreshadowed the modern wear and tear theorists when he asserted: "much exercise and weariness consumes the spirits and substances." Sustained and straining effort in any direction, whether it be mental or physical, cannot be continued without a following train of troubles. When any function of the body is put in action there is a chemical change within the tissues which gives rise to the energy set free, and before new power may be had the substance which affords this energy must be rebuilt. While this is true of all the tissues of the body, owing to the greater bulk of the muscular system the changes are apparently more active in this organism. Tire is recognized more speedily, while incessant activity often prevents an adequate opportunity for repair.

We have seen that the Incas, during the period when their young men were preparing for knighthood, devot-

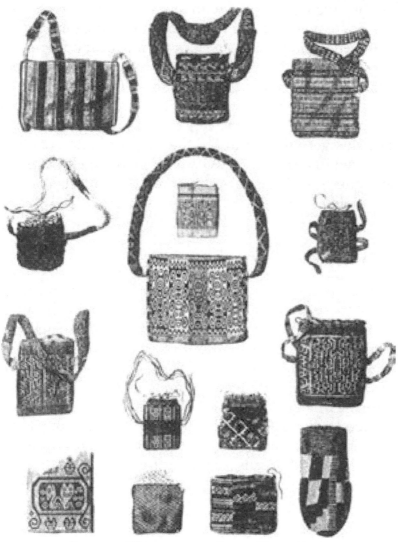

*Incan Chuspas—Coca Pouches*

ed the greatest attention  to athletic training.  It was only
when the young nobles had proved themselves worthy,
by appropriate exhibition of their powers of endurance,
that they were presented with the *chuspa* in which to carry
the Coca leaves, and the *poporo* to contain the lime to be
employed in preparing the Coca for mastication. These
decorations were thereafter worn through life as emblems
of ennoblement, and buried with the mummied body, the
Coca affording support on the journey to the unknown.
The ancient philosophers were quite as ignorant of the
exact changes which induced the transformation of energy
displayed in muscular activity as were the Incas, or as are
the modern Andeans regarding the true workings of Coca
in its yield of force.

# Structure of Muscle

The muscular system comprises two varieties of muscles.
One of these acts under mental influence, while the other
acts independent of the will, while the heart—which is
essentially a muscle-—partakes of qualities in both of these
varieties. The voluntary muscles are chiefly attached to the
bony framework, and are concerned in bodily movements,
while the involuntary muscles enter into the formation of
the blood vessels, the lymphatics and the walls of various
structures, as the air passages, the alimentary canal and
other important organs, as well as forming parts of the skin
and mucous membranes.

The framework muscles are supported by thin sheaths
of tissue, which in their interior divide by numerous ram-
ifications and separate the contained muscular substance
into bundles. These are still further divided into little
fibres, each ultimate fibre being enveloped with a close
network of minute blood vessels. These vessels afford an
ample means for bringing nutriment to the muscle substance, as well as for carrying away the waste products

which are constantly being formed, even in the state commonly regarded as absolute rest. The importance of this hurrying stream of nutriment, and waste elimination to the muscular organism, may be inferred from the estimate that one-fourth of the entire blood of the body is contained in the muscles.

When the little muscle fibres are examined under the microscope, they are seen to be made up of alternating lines which appear as light and dark striations. The darker of these lines, when viewed in transverse section, is found composed of little polygonal compartments. Within these divisions is contained a semi-fluid material which has been demonstrated to be the contractile element of the muscle substance.

The ancients presumed the muscles acted by some pulling influence exerted through the nerves. Harmonious nerve action is essential to every movement, yet muscle substance has been shown to have an inherent property of contractility quite independent of nerve influence. The chief nerves controlling the movements of the muscular system have their origin in the brain and spinal cord. These each consist of fibres conveying sensation and fibres which control motion. These latter end in expansions on the surface of the muscle in intimate contact with the contractile element, the function of which it regulates through the reflex influence of the sensory nerves. In other words a stimulation of the sensory nerves excites the motor nerves to cause muscular activity.

Each fibre is not continuous through the entire length of muscle structure, but the tapering end of one fibre is united to the body of its neighbor by a cement-like substance to form a bundle which constitutes the muscle proper. These bundles taper, or are expanded, as the case may be, to a dense fibrous tissue for attachment to different portions of the movable framework of the body. When a muscle acts, each of its individual fibres shortens through some chemical influence of the contractile element. The combined action of the fibres exerts a pull toward either end of the muscle, which occasions movement of the less fixed portion of the framework to which the muscle is attached.

The involuntary muscles have not definite tendons like the voluntary muscles, and their microscopical structure is also different, their fibres being smaller and instead of being cross-striped they are marked longitudinally. In their arrangement the fibres are so interlaced that by their contraction they lessen the capacity of the vessels or organs in the walls of which they are located.

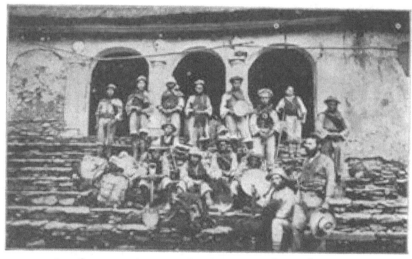

*Andean miners sitting on church steps*

The property of contraction is inherent in the muscle itself, and continues even after its nerve supply has been cut off. For this experiment in the laboratory, curare is employed; this paralyzes the nerve filaments deep down in the muscle substance yet leaves the muscle intact. Under these conditions though contraction will not be produced when the nerve is stimulated, movement will follow when stimulus is directly applied to the muscle substance. It is presumed that this inherent property is generated by some substance brought in the blood, which induces a chemical change in the contractile element and liberates the energy displayed as muscular movement. This change is influenced by temperature, and by the presence or absence of waste material in the muscle structure or in the circulation. Whatever this explosive substance may be, it is presumed to be built up in the muscle structure from some carbohydrate material—possibly glycogen—under the influence of a nitrogenous substance. For, as Foster has said: "The whole secret of life may almost be said to be wrapped up in the occult properties of certain nitrogen compounds." Hermann named this hypothetical substance inogen.

During a muscle contraction it is inferred this carbohydrate splits into carbonic acid, sarcolactic acid and some nitrogenous material which may be myosin or a substance akin to it, the acids being carried off in the blood stream, while the proteid substance remains in the muscle to be again elaborated into the inogen energy yielding material. Helmholtz calculated that in the human body one-fifth the energy of the material consumed goes out as work, thus contrasting favorably with the steam engine, in which it hardly ever amounts to more than one-tenth.

According to the theory of Liebig the nitrogenous food is utilized in the building up of proteid tissues, and the non-nitrogenous food is exclusively devoted to heat producing purposes, being directly oxidized in the blood, while its excess is stored as fat. In accordance with this theory, muscular exercise increases the waste of muscle substance, while the wear and tear is estimated by the amount of urea excreted. Originally this idea was generally accepted, but was attacked from many sources when it was found that facts of subsequent research did not coincide. Troube suggested in opposition that muscle and nerve tissue is not destroyed by exercise, but that force is contributed to these tissues through the oxidation of non-nitrogenous substances of which the muscle and nerve were simply mediums of expression.

# Exercise

Following the idea of Liebig, that work results in wear and tear of the tissues, there should be an increased output of nitrogen during exertion, but many observers in trying to harmonize results with this view have found little increase of urea—which practically represents all the nitrogen passed out of the body—while a decided increase of urea is found from the consumption of nitrogenous foods. Among the more noted experiments which controverted the theory that the nitrogenous waste represented the relative expenditure of energy is that of Dr. Fick, Professor of Physiology, and Dr. "Wislicenus, Professor of Chemistry, both of the University of Zurich. They ascended the Faulhorn, two thousand metres high (6,561 feet) for the purpose of determining the resultant wear and tear upon the nitrogenous tissues from a known amount of exercise.

To accurately determine this, they limited their diet to non-nitrogenous materials, taking starch, fat and a little sugar, with beer, wine and tea as beverages. For seventeen hours before the ascent they limited themselves to non-nitrogenous food, and their first examinations were made eleven hours before their start. The ascent was completed in eight hours, and after a rest of six hours they ate an ordinary meal, which included meat. The urine secreted was examined to estimate the nitrogen excreted for. each hour's work, which showed the following results:

### Nitrogen Excreted Per House in Grammes

| | | |
|---|---|---|
| Before work ..................... | 0.63 | 0.61 |
| Work................................ | 0.41 | 0.39 |
| After work. . ..................... | 0.40 | 0.40 |
| Night................................ | 0.45 | 0.51 |

This indicates that the amount of nitrogen excreted was in relation to the food eaten and not to the work done, less relative nitrogen being passed in the "work" and "after work" periods when on a non-nitrogenous diet than during the period when nitrogenous food was eaten. The calculations were based on the amount of work which the oxidation of muscular substance containing fifteen per cent, of nitrogen would produce as determined from the excreted urea. The result showed this inadequate to have enabled the experimenters to perform the task which they did, Fick's work exceeding the theoretical amount by one-half, while that done by Wislicenus was in excess by more

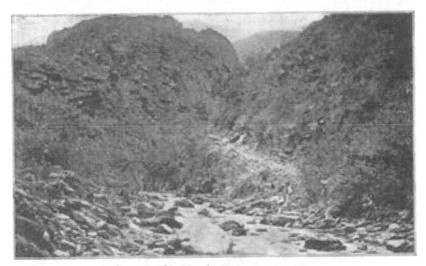

*The Puli-Puli River in Peru*

than three-fourths the theoretical amount, without in either case considering the necessary work of the various vital processes. These facts led many experimenters to further investigation, and resulted in a decided reaction from Liebig's rigid theory, which had been accepted more literally than that physiologist intended. Instead of regarding the decomposition of proteids as the sole source of muscular energy, the carbohydrates were now looked upon as a formative element for generating force, because during muscular activity the glycogen stored in muscle disappears, to accumulate again during rest.

Pfliiger, one of the most eminent of modern physiologists, in attempting to harmonize the theory of Liebig, experimented with a dog, which he kept upon an exclusive meat diet free from fat, and made him perform hard labor several times a day for weeks, during which the animal showed: "Very extraordinary strength and elasticity in all his movements." In this experiment he wished to show that all the energy produced during hard work was from the transformation of proteid. To further show whether proteid simply was compensatory, he gave a mixed diet, and this led him to the conclusion that in a diet composed of proteid, carbohydrates and fats the quantity of the two latter substances destroyed in metabolism depends wholly upon the fact whether much or little proteid be fed. His conclusions are that: "In general the quantity of carbohydrates and fat that undergoes destruction is smaller the greater the income of proteid." This may be regarded as the accepted view of modern physiologists with this qualification, that proteids must be built up from carbohydrates under a nitrogenous stimulus, just as we have Been is the process in plant structure.

It has already been pointed out that the nitrogenous Coca has a direct bearing upon the structure of tissue through a possible quality of elaborating the carbohydrates of the protoplasm into proteids. Since the muscles form the largest bulk of tissues in the body in which chemical changes are constantly going on, it may be inferred how important is this upbuilding of the complex substance by which muscle activity is produced. The action of Coca on yeast as well as penicillium and other low organisms indicates its peculiar activity upon protoplasm. The experiments of Huxley and Martin long since showed that penicillium can build itself up out of ammonium tartrate and inorganic salts, and can by a decomposition of itself give rise to fats and other bodies, and we have every reason, says Foster, to suppose this constructive power belongs naturally to all native protoplasm wherever found. At the same time we see, even in the case of penicillium, it is of advantage to offer to the protoplasm as food, substances which are on their way to become protoplasm, which thus saves the organism much constructive labor. "It is not unreasonable, even if opposed to established ideas, to suppose that the animal protoplasm is as constructive as the vegetable protoplasm, the difference between the two being that the former, unlike the latter, is as destructive as it is constructive, and therefore requires to be continually fed with ready constructed material."

In further support of the influence of Coca upon the formation of proteid it may be again emphasized that the nitrogen found in the urea is not a measure of the proteid transformation of the body. This conclusion would be justified if it were known that all nitrogenous cleavage products of the proteid molecule without exception leave the body. But there is no ground for such belief. On the contrary, there is no fact known to contradict the idea that nitrogenous cleavage products of the proteid molecule can rebuild themselves synthetically again into proteid with the aid of new non-nitrogenous groups of atoms. This latter possibility has been overlooked, and in consequence views have arisen, especially in relation to muscle metabolism, which though bearing the stamp of improbability have been accepted and handed down, but which recently have been criticised by Pfliiger.

Just where urea is manufactured in the organism is not definitely known. It is presumed that *kreatin, xanthin* and other nitrogenous extractives which are found in the circulation resulting from tissue activity may be converted either by the blood or by the epithelium of the kidneys, and discharged as urea. In certain kidney diseases it is known that these waste products are retained in the circulation, with consequent symptoms of poisoning. In addition to this it has been found that an increase of nitrogenous food rapidly augments this excretion, the products of intestinal digestion, the *leucin* and *tyrosin,* being carried to the liver and converted by the liver cells to urea, and this organ is considered at least the chief organ of urea formation.

# Protoplasm

It has been found that in functional derangements of the liver, when the normal urea formation is interfered with, there is imperfect oxidation of the products which should be eliminated as urea, and a deposit of lithates occurs in the urine as a signal of imperfect oxidation. This also may follow excessive exercise. In serious organic diseases the urea excretion may cease entirely, being replaced by the less oxidized *leucin* and *tyrosin.* M. Genevoix, from observations of his own and those of Charcot, Bouchardat and others, concludes that disorders of the liver which do not seriously implicate the secreting structure of that tissue increase the amount of urea excreted, while graver disorders diminish it very considerably. A Belgian physician, Doctor Kommel-aere, maintains that diagnosis of cancer of the stomach may be made when the urea excretion falls and continues below ten grammes a day for several consecutive days.

The average excretion of urea is sixteen grains an hour, the excretion fluctuating between thirteen and twenty-five grains, being greater soon after eating, and much less during the early morning hours. Uric acid, which is probably a less advanced form of oxidation, being present in the relation to urea as one to thirty-five, its relation to body weight being three and a half grains per pound; thus when urea excretion equals thirty-five grains for each ten pounds of body weight, there is commonly present one grain of uric acid. The effect of these waste products in the tissues is to so impede the functions of the cells as to occasion symptoms of depression and fatigue, whether this be manifested by irritability, drowsiness or profound muscular tire. There is a loading up—not necessarily within the cells of the tissues, but in the blood stream which supplies these—of excreta which vitiates the proper pabulum of the protoplasm, and a period of rest is absolutely necessary to enable the tissues to get rid of this matter before a healthful condition may be resumed.

All the symptoms of fatigue are due to the effort of the tissues at repair. There is an increase of respiration to bring the necessary increase of oxygen demanded, and accompanying this respiratory effort there is a frequency of the heart beat, while the body becomes cool because its heat is lessened through the evaporation of perspiration. In protracted fatigue there may be a rise of temperature due to irritation by the increased force of the blood stream, occasioning sleeplessness, while the digestive functions are interfered with because of the excessive demands of other organs on the blood stimulus.

## Cause of Fatigue

In over exertion, where there is actual loss of proteid tissue, the effects of prostration and tire may not be experienced immediately, but only after several days. Simiļlar symptoms to these accompany the infectious diseases when the blood is loaded with the products formed by invading bacteria. Again they are manifest when the organism is poisoned through toxic products of indigestion. These may be simply the products of proteid decomposition—*leucomaines* as they are termed, or they may be *ptomaines* produced by the activity of certain micro-organisms which affect the body through the toxic principles which they elaborate. Some of these are excessively poisonous in minute doses, and are chiefly developed in such articles of food as milk,

ice cream, cheese, sausage and canned fish. It has been inferred that the muscles may also produce toxins which by
their presence give rise to poisonous symptoms.

From whatever source they may have been derived,
waste products in the blood impede the action of all the
tissues of the body. This influence is well shown in the
laboratory upon a prepared muscle, the contractions being
recorded by a series of curves upon a suitable machine.

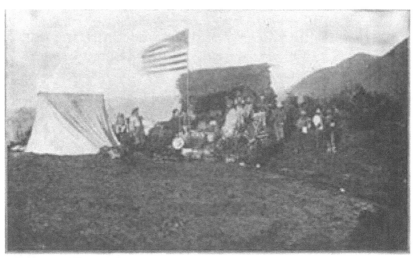

*Camp of Explorers Between Phara and Aporoma.*

Following stimulation there is a short interval known as
the latent period, and then contraction is indicated by a
rising curve commencing rapidly and proceeding more
slowly to a maximum height, and as the muscle returns to
its normal condition there is a descending curve, at first
sudden and then more gradual. After repeated shocks of
stimulation these curves become less marked, until the
contractions record almost a continuous line—a condition
which is termed muscular tetanus.

Such tired muscle has a longer latent period than a
fresh one, and a stronger stimulation is necessary to produce contractions equal to those at the beginning of exper-

imentation. Bernard experimented with blue bottle flies—
*musca vomi-toria,* and found that the muscle of fatigued
flies compared with that of flies at rest showed microscopical distinction, the contractile disks of the tired muscle being almost obliterated, while the capacity of such a muscle
for taking a stain for microscopic examination evidenced
an important difference over that of normal muscle, the
whole contents of the segments staining uniformly, indicating that extraordinary exertion had used up the muscular
substance more rapidly than it was repaired.

Ranke found that by washing out a fatigued muscle
with common salt solution, though it added no new factor
of energy, it freed the tissue from poisonous excreta and
enabled it to again perform work. To confirm this a watery
extract of fatigued muscle, when injected into fresh muscle,
occasioned it to lose its working capacity. Mosso has also
shown by experiments on the dog the presence of these
fatigue substances. When the blood of a tired dog was
injected into a dog which had been at rest all the phenomena of fatigue were manifest, but when the blood injected
was from a normally resting dog no such symptoms were
induced. This physiologist has shown that in man small
doses of cocaine remove the fatigue sense and raise muscular ability above normal.

Dr. Alexander Haig, of London, attributes all the symptoms of depression and fatigue as due to the presence of
uric acid in the blood, which he regards as the particular
poison of the excreta. Uric acid, he claims, obstructs the
capillaries throughout the entire body, the consequent defi-
cient circulation preventing a proper metabolism by retarding the removal of waste products.

The relative excretion of waste is influenced not only
by the routine of living, but by changes in the weather, tire
being more easily produced in warm than in cold weather
because of the increased elimination of acids by perspiration raising the alkalinity of the blood and permitting the

passage of an excess of uric acid from the tissues into the blood. With this excess there is a diminished excretion of urea accompanied by the symptoms of fatigue. Exercise when excessive increases the formation of urea, which may at first be carried off in a free blood stream, but when the flow in the capillaries is diminished through the presence of uric acid in excess, the urea excretion is retarded and fatigue is manifest.

Cocaine, it is found, will free the blood of uric acid and abolish all the symptoms of fatigue both of mind and body, doing this by raising the acidity of the blood and so directly counteracting the effect of exercise by preventing the blood becoming a solvent for uric acid. The effect of the pure blood is to produce a free circulation with increased metabolism in the muscles and nerve centres. When the blood is loaded with excreta the circulation is retarded and there is high blood pressure, which may ultimately result in dilatation of the heart.

The long train of troubles which may follow retention of waste have been found to be worse during the morning hours when the acid tide of the urine is lowest. These conditions are all relieved under the influence of Coca, a knowledge of which has been gleaned from its empirical use. As an instance of this, a lady suffering from a severe influenza accompanied with rheumatism, was induced to try a grog of Vin Mariani—as advocated by Dr. Cyrus Edson in the treatment of La Grippe, and much to her surprise found that she was not only cured of her cold, but entirely relieved from the symptoms of her rheumatism as well, despite a preformed prejudice against Coca in any form. Acting upon this suggestive hint, I have found that alternate doses of Coca and the salicylates constitute an admirable treatment for rheumatism.

# Sustenance with Coca

The influence of Coca in banishing the effects of extreme fatigue is well illustrated in an account of its use communicated to me by Dr. Frank L. James, Editor of the *National Druggist*, St. Louis. While a student at Munich he experimented with the use of Coca upon himself at the request of Professor Liebig, whose pupil he was. On one occasion, when exceedingly tired both physically and mentally, he was induced to try chewing Coca after the proper Peruvian fashion with a little *llipta*. Before commencing this experiment he was hungry, but too tired to eat and too hungry to sleep. In a few moments after beginning to chew hunger gave place to a sense of warmth in the stomach, while all physical weariness disappeared, though mentally he was still somewhat tired and disinclined to read or study, though this condition soon passed away, giving rise to an absolute eagerness to be at some sort of exercise. These sensations lasted altogether for probably three hours, gradually passing off after the first hour, leaving the subject none the worse for his experience and able to eat a hearty dinner the same evening.

Some years afterward, while practicing in the South, this gentleman returned from a thirty-six hours' ride so tired as to necessitate being helped off the horse and upstairs to his room. While preparing for bed his eyes fell upon a package of Coca leaves which he had recently received by way of San Francisco, and the idea immediately occurred to him to repeat the experiment of his student days. In the course of a quarter of an hour—following the chewing of probably a drachm of Coca leaves—he felt so refreshed and recuperated that he was able to go out and visit patients about the town to whom he had previously sent word that he was too tired to call on them that night. In describing the result, Dr. James said: "I was not very hungry at the time before taking the Coca, but all sense of the necessity or of a desire for food vanished with the weariness."

Professor Novy, of the University of Michigan, is referred to by one of his former classmates as having formed one of a group of experimenters upon the vise of Coca leaves. The influence being tested during a walk of twenty-four miles, taken one afternoon without any other nourishment but water and Coca. Over four miles an hour was averaged, and although unaccustomed to such long walks or vigorous exercise, no special muscular fatigue was experienced by four of the party who chewed the leaves almost constantly during the journey. No change was noted in the urine and no depression was experienced the next day. One who did not chew Coca, but was addicted to alcohol and chewed tobacco constantly, was somewhat more fatigued than the others, and suffered considerably from soreness of the muscles on the following day.

The experience of Sir Robert Christison, of Edinburgh, with the use of Coca upon himself and several of his stu-

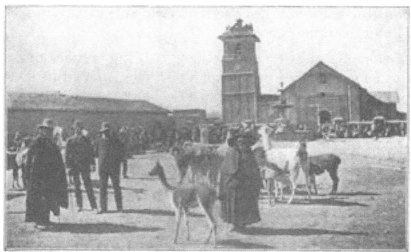

*Plaza and Church at Azangaro, Peru.*
*The inside walls of the church are covered*
*with sheets of gold.*

dents, is full of interest because of his extended experiments and the high rank of the investigator. Two of his students, unaccustomed to exercise during five months, walked some sixteen miles without having eaten any food since breakfast. On their return they each took two drachms of Coca made into an infusion, to which was added five grains of carbonate of soda, in imitation of the Peruvian method of adding an alkali. All sense of hunger and fatigue soon left, and after an hour's walk they returned to enjoy an excellent dinner, after which they felt alert during the evening, and their night's sleep was sound and refreshing. One of these students felt a slight sensation of giddiness after drinking the infusion, but the other experienced no unpleasant symptoms. Ten students, under similar conditions, walked varying distances, from twenty to thirty miles, over a hilly road.

Two of these were unable to remark any effects from the use of Coca, several felt decided relief from fatigue, while four experienced complete relief, and one of these had walked thirty miles without any food. Professor Christison, though seventy-eight years of age and unaccustomed to vigorous exercise, subsequently experimented on himself by chewing Coca leaves with and without *llipta,* some of which had been forwarded to him from Peru. He first determined the effect of profound fatigue by walking fifteen miles on two occasions without taking food or drink. On his return his pulse, which was normally sixty-two at rest, was one hundred and ten on his arrival home, and two hours later was ninety. He was unfit for mental work in the evening, though he slept soundly all night, but the next morning was not inclined for active exercise.

Then, under similar conditions, he walked sixteen miles, in three stages of four, six, and six miles, with one interval of half an hour, and two intervals of an hour and a half. During the last forty-five minutes of his second rest he chewed eighty grains of Coca, reserving forty grains for use during the last stage, even swallowing some of the fibre. He felt sufficiently tired to look forward to the end of his journey with reluctance, and did not observe any particular effect from the Coca until he got out of doors and put on his usual pace, of which he said: "At once I was surprised to find that all sense of weariness had entirely fled and that I could proceed not only with ease, but even with elasticity. I got over the six miles in an hour and a half without difficulty, and found it easy when done to get up a four and a half mile pace and to ascend quickly two steps at a time to my dressing room, two floors up-stairs; in short, I had no sense of fatigue or any other uneasiness whatsoever."

During this walk he perspired profusely. On reaching home his pulse was ninety, and in two hours it had fallen to seventy-two, showing that the heart and circulation had been strengthened under the influence of Coca. The urine solids were the same as during the walk without Coca. In describing this walk, he said: "On arrival home before dinner, I felt neither hunger nor thirst, after complete abstinence from food and drink of every kind for nine hours, but upon dinner appearing in half an hour, ample justice was done to it." After a sound sleep through the night he woke refreshed and free from all sense of fatigue.

An influence of Coca not anticipated was the relief of a tenderness of his eyes, which during some years had rendered continuous reading a painful effort. In another trial at mountain climbing, he ascended Ben Vorlieh, on Loch Earn, 3,224 feet above the sea. The climb was along a rugged foot path, then through a short heather and deep grass, and the final dome of seven hundred feet rise was among blocks and slabs of mica-slate. The ascent was made in two and a half hours, the last three hundred feet requiring considerable determination.

His companions enjoyed a luncheon, but Sir Robert contented himself chewing two-thirds of a drachm of Coca, and after a rest of three-quarters of an hour was ready for the descent. Al-

*The chewing of Coca not only removes extreme fatigue, but prevents it. Hunger and thirst are suspended, but eventually appetite and digestion are unaffected. No injury whatever is sustained at the time or subsequently in occasional trials.*

though this was looked forward to with no little distrust, he found upon rising that all fatigue was gone, and he journeyed with the same ease with which he had enjoyed mountain rambles in his youth. The experimenter was neither weary, hungry nor thirsty, and felt as though he could easily have walked four miles to his home. After a hearty dinner, followed by a busy evening, he slept soundly during the night and woke refreshed in the morning, ready for another day's exercise.

During the trip he took neither food nor drink of any kind except chewing sixty grains of Coca leaves. Eight days after this experiment was repeated, using ninety grains of Coca. The weather had changed and the temperature was forty-four degrees at the top of the mountain and a chilly breeze provoked the desire to descend. While resting sixty grains of Coca was chewed. The descent was made without halt in an hour and a quarter, and followed by a walk of two miles over a level road to meet his carriage. He then felt slightly tired, because three hours had elapsed since he had chewed Coca.

In summing up his experience Professor Christison says: "I feel that without details the general results which may now be summarized would scarcely carry conviction with them. They are the following: The chewing of Coca not only removes extreme fatigue, but prevents it. Hunger and thirst are suspended, but eventually appetite and di-

gestion are unaffected. No injury whatever is sustained at
the time or subsequently in occasional trials." From sixty to
ninety grains are sufficient for one trial, but some persons
either require more or are constitutionally proof against
the restorative action of Coca. From his observations there
was no effect on the mental faculties except to prevent the
dullness and drowsiness which follow great bodily fatigue.

It is a matter of much interest to determine just what
food is appropriate to generate muscle or to stimulate the
tissues for work. As the capacity of an organ is in proportion to its bulk—under proper conditions—it seems
essential that proteids should be eaten in order to create
the muscle substances of which they form so great a part;
but as has been repeatedly indicated, no one variety of
food makes that same variety of tissue. All conversion in
the body is due to a chemical change within the cell of the
tissue; the food taken in is broken down by the digestive
processes, and after assimilation is doled out according
to the particular requirements of the individual parts of a
normal organism.

The muscles are not set at work from the immediate
intake of food, but are rendered capable for action by a
chemical conversion of the material already stored up in
the tissues, which is elaborated into energy as it may be
required. It would seem as though this fact had not been
carefully considered when calculating the effect of any diet
upon muscular exertion during a brief period. The capacity
of the body for work is due to the integrity of its tissue and
the ability to draw suitable supplies from these stored substances. It is the appropriate conversion of this stored-up
material which constitutes energy in a capable being rather
than a mere automatism. Without this power of conversion
the human organism would simply be clogged up by an
accumulation of fuel which would impede rather than create activity. The body should not be regarded as a machine
constituted with certain working parts which are gradually

worn out through the so often expressed "wear and tear." The facts long since have proved that life is a succession of deaths. The highest type of physical life is that which is capable of the greatest activity, creating useful energy and properly eliminating the waste matters resulting from the chemical changes from this conversion. Indeed, one of the gravest problems in the maintenance of a healthful activity is the one of excretion. To the retention of waste products in the blood or tissues a whole train of ills, both physical and mental, is unquestionably due, whether this poison be uric acid or not.

Preoccupied humanity seems constantly seeking some medicinal measure toward buoyancy and vigor rather than regarding the rational effects of appropriate eating and proper exercise. The success of many patent nostrums is chiefly based upon the fact of the necessity for elimination, and a good diuretic or laxative disguised as a panacea for all ills often produces the required result. As to the proper food essential to promote the greatest energy there have been many conflicting conclusions drawn from the known physiological facts.

On the one side it has been asserted that all energy is induced from nitrogenous substances, while on the other side equally competent observers have asserted that the non-nitrogenous substances are alone used; yet all the evidence points to the fact that the constructive metabolism in animals is paralleled by similar processes in plant life, in which it has been shown that carbohydrates are built up into proteids, while these latter are also broken down into carbohydrates, and each of these may be converted again and again under the appro-

*Humanity seems constantly seeking some medicinal measure toward buoyancy and vigor rather than regarding the rational effects of appropriate eating and proper exercise.*

priate stimulus of the other substance. We know that starch, which is the representative of the carbohydrate class, is converted into glucose and carried to the liver to be stored up as the animal starch—glycogen—and as the various tissues of the body are called into activity this stored-up material is hurried to them in a soluble form to be utilized by the cell in the production of energy. When meat is eaten—which is the representative type of the nitrogenous class—its proteid material is changed into a soluble peptone, and this, carried to the liver, is converted into glycogen, which indicates, as has been proven by experiment, that either class of food substance is capable of maintaining the functions of the body so long as the chemical elements comprising the food taken be appropriate. While the meat eater and the vegetarian are each right, they are equally both wrong when advocating an exclusiveness in either dietary. The fact is, as will be shown in the chapter upon dietetics, it is purely an individual matter as to what particular food may be best. It all depends upon the body, or the machine—as you will—as to what substance each particular organism shall have the privilege of converting into energy.

## Appropriate Dietary

While the body may be supported on either class of foodstuffs for a time, a man would surely starve as quick on a purely nitrogenous dietary as he would upon one purely non-nitrogenous. It will be recalled that the experiment of Fick and Wislicenus was conducted upon a food, the solid portion of which was carbohydrate, but with this tea was drunk as a beverage. Tea loaded with xanthin would afford sufficient of the nitrogenous element to convert the stored-up carbohydrates to action, but as Haig and Morton have both shown, tea contains so much of an equivalent to uric acid that it could not long be relied upon as an energy exciter, for while the tissue might be stimulated for a time, waste matter would soon be augmented in the blood. Coca, as we have seen, has the quality of freeing the blood from waste material, and yet possesses sufficient nitrogenous quality to convert the stored-up carbohydrates into tissue and energy. The Andeans are a race small of stature and of low muscular development. The average American or European could easily tire a native Indian in a day's travel, but while the former continuing on an ordinary diet would soon become stiff the Indian sustained by Coca remains fit and active, and is apparently fresh and ready after a hard day's jaunt. It seems probable that this condition is occasioned through the converting influence of the nitrogenous Coca acting upon the stored-up carbohydrates of the Andean's accustomed dietary. Thus while promoting metabolism and increasing energy the blood current is at the same time kept free.

The custom of the Andean to measure distances by the *cocada* has already been referred to; it is the length of time that the influence of a chew of Coca will carry him—equal to a period of some forty minutes—and during which he will cover nearly two miles on a level ground or a mile and a quarter up hill. Taking the suggestion from this a preparation of Coca made in Paris known as "Velo-Coca," is purposely intended for the use of bicyclists, a given dose of which is calculated to sustain the rider through forty kilometres—twenty-five miles. The advantage of Coca in long distance contests has long been known to certain professionals, who have endeavored to keep their use of this force sustainer a secret.

PAINTING REPRESENTING SUN WORSHIP, FROM A VASE AT CUZCO.  [*Wiener.*]

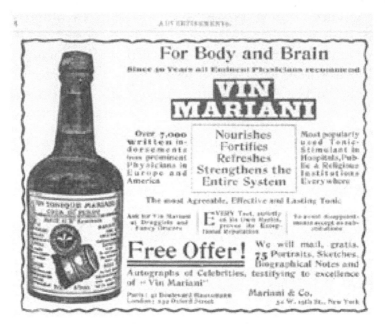

Some years ago the members of the Toronto La Crosse Club experimented with Coca, and during the season when that club held the championship of the world Coca was used in all its important matches. The Toronto Club was composed of men accustomed to sedentary work, while some of the opposing players were sturdy men accustomed to out of door exercise. The games were all very severely contested, and some were played in the hottest weather of one summer; on one occasion the thermometer registered 110° F. in the sun.

The more stalwart appearing men, however, were so far used up before the match was completed that they could hardly be encouraged to finish the concluding game, "while the Coca chewers were as elastic and apparently as free from fatigue as at the commencement of the play." At the beginning of the game each player was given from one drachm to a drachm and a half of leaves, and this amount, without lime or any other addition, was chewed in small portions during the game. The first influence experienced was a dryness of the throat, which, when relieved by gargling with water, was not again noticed, while a sense of invigoration and an increase of muscular force was soon experienced, and this continued through the game, so that fatigue was resisted. The pulse was increased in frequency and perspiration was excited, but no mental symptoms were induced excepting an exhilaration of spirits, which was not followed by any after effects.

As has been shown, fatigue and its ills is occasioned by a diminution of the elements necessary to activity as well as to an excess of waste materials in the blood. This latter cause alone explains many problems dependent upon this condition which are commonly assigned to other causes. Under this hypothesis it is easy to appreciate not only the cause of muscle fatigue, but the irritability from nerve tire as well as the restlessness in wasting disease. When the tissues are not supplied with a blood stream that is pure and uncontaminated they cannot respond healthfully. A blood current already overburdened with waste can neither stimulate to activity nor carry off the burden of excreta.

The power of Coca to relieve the circulation, and so bring about a condition indicating a free blood stream, has been emphasized by a host of observers. Speaking of the action of but one of its alkaloids, Dr. Haig says: "Some have asserted that it is oblivion men seek for when they take opium, cocaine, etc., I believe this to be a great error. Give me an eternity of oblivion and I would exchange it for one hour with my cerebral circulation quite free from uric acid, and opium or cocaine will free it for me. When the blood stream is free the pulse tension is reduced, the rate is quickened, and the increased flow alters the mental condition as if by magic; ideas flash through the brain; everything is remembered."

Hitherto the usual explanation that has been advanced as to the influence of Coca—when any influence has been accorded—has been its stimulant action upon the nerves. In view of the facts set forth in this research such a theory

seems inadequate. I have endeavored to show by a succession of facts and many examples, that the sustaining
influence of Coca in fatigue, as well as its curative power
in so many diseased conditions, as to render it a seeming
panacea, is largely due to a direct action upon the cells of
the tissues, as well as through the property which Coca has
of freeing the blood from waste.

This influence may chiefly be upon the brain or upon
the muscular structure, in accordance with the relative proportion of the associate principles present in the Coca leaf
employed. Under this hypothesis, based upon physiological research as well as upon the theory of the formation of
proteid in plants and in animals, Coca not only stimulates
the cells to activity and so sets free energy, but may build
up new tissue through exciting the protoplasm to appropriate conversion. Such an hypothesis is certainly plausible
when we consider the action of amides and other nitrogenous elements in plant structure. This is again emphasized
by its harmony with recent theories of Pfliiger regarding
the building up of proteid tissue in the animal organism.
So much testimony points to this conclusion that in the entire absence of other scientific explanation this is certainly
worthy of serious consideration. The facts of which will be
more specifically elaborated in the chapter on physiology.

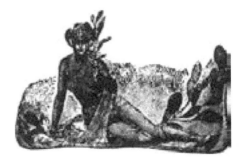

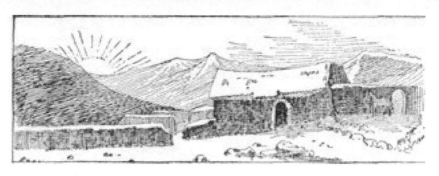

# Chapter 7

# Action on the Nervous System

E may presume an ideal condition of health, but there is no practical standard by which this can be gauged. Each individual organism presents a maximum and minimum range of vigor, between which the true balance must lie for that one being. The powers of the aboriginal Indian, while of a different quality, were not necessarily of a higher type than are those of the nervous worker of today, nor was the life of the former necessarily more natural because more active. We are creatures of the circumstances and environments in which cast. Each condition must be compared with its class. The possibilities of combating severe disease are vastly superior under the results of modern civilization. Man in every age must maintain a balance amidst the peculiar environment to which he is subjected, and the result of progress is to develop hygienic resources as well as keener susceptibilities.

The functions of the body are governed through the action of the nervous system involuntarily, whether the subject be asleep or awake, in sickness or in health. This action, however, may be influenced by the will either to depress or excite individual functions, so that their action may be modified or even perverted to a condition of disease. Dr. John Hunter, who was a victim to his own emotions, emphasized this when he wrote: "Every part of the body sympathizes with the mind, for whatever affects the mind, the body is affected in proportion."

Among the annoyances incidental to a modern civilization are those troubles produced from a possible nervous perversion, engendered through overtaxing the powers mentally or physically in the modern whirl and bustle of a busy life. We all realize the effects of muscular fatigue, but few seem to appreciate the extreme tire, which is possible to the nervous system of the purely sedentary worker. This may manifest itself in the mildest form as a mere irritability or restlessness, or more profoundly as peevishness and even despondency.

It is not as easy to demonstrate nerve tire in the laboratory as it is to show the fatigue of muscle, yet there can be no doubt that similar factors are at work to induce either. It is known that all the activity of the tissues, of whatever kind, is due to a chemical conversion of the substance contained in the minute cells which go to complete the organism. Fatigue results from the retention of products of waste in the blood which normally should be excreted. As a result the tissues are not properly nourished by a purified circulation for their work, and exhaustion is a consequence, whether the structure under this influence be muscle or nerve.

When we learn that Coca relieves muscular tire, mental depression or nervous fatigue, that it calms to refreshing sleep or stimulates to wakefulness and activity, that it allays hunger or induces appetite as the case may be, we can only harmonize such seemingly opposite applications through appreciating that this influence is extended to the tissues through the fluid which supplies them with nourishment. We have already seen that the blood is so speedily purified under the action of Coca that the circulation may at once return an appropriate pabulum to all the cells of the body and so may promote in them a normally healthful action.

The brain may be broadly considered as made up of cells and nerve fibres. The outer portion, which is termed the cortex, consists of many convolutions which through this arrangement affords a greater superficial area for the brain cells. These cells are located in layers over the surface, as well as arranged in groups at the base of the brain and in the medulla and spinal cord. The convolutions are merely rudimentary in animals and are poorly developed in the lower orders of the human race and in the uneducated. By intellectual development these are increased in a manner quite analogous to that in which muscle is increased by exercise. Gross bulk of brain substance does not necessarily indicate giant intellect, but merely the structure for such possible development.

# Intellectual Development

The brain practically attains its greatest size in early childhood, at least this is the period of its most active increase, and remembering the law that the part of the body which is subject to the greatest physiological growth is most liable to disease, it will keep before us the fact that children are particularly susceptible to disorders of the brain and nervous system. In childhood the tendency should be to restrain these organs, which are already too alert, from an undue excitement.

From birth an education of the individual cells of this intellectual centre should be carefully conducted. A refinement of nerve tissue progressing by easy gradations until strength and power shall be secured. It is through this alone that man may be raised superior to the beast or savage. Not only present enjoyments but future comforts and realizations are so absolutely dependent upon this that even "Spiritual life can only reach the human form by and through the brain cell."

Quite as important as the brain in maintaining mental stability is the action of the sympathetic nerve in controlling physical well being, while both brain and sympathetic nerve must act together to sustain the organism in true harmony. The sympathetic nerve runs on either side and in front of the spinal column as a double chain of little brains. From these centers not only the great organs are supplied, but also the coats of the blood vessels, through which association a controlling influence is maintained over the entire organism. Along its route these nerves are intimately connected with branch nerve fibres from the brain and spinal cord. Through groups of fibres sent to the heart, to the stomach and to the organs of the pelvis the functions of either one of these may be influenced in sympathy from the derangement of some other organ far distant, the workings of which are not directly associated, but the action of which is affected by a reflection of the troubles elsewhere. This reflex effect between distant parts of the body is analogous to the switching on of a branch telegraph loop to the main line to carry news to points with which it was not directly connected.

So intimate is the relation of this regulating nerve with the various functions of the body that it is possible for these to be seriously interfered with through action of the sympathetic on the blood vessels, by which the tension of their walls is altered and the circulation is accordingly hastened or retarded. Common examples of this effect are seen when the emotions are excited and occasion the capillary vessels to contract as in pallor, or, when these are suddenly dilated, to cause blushing. The idea that the emotions have their seat in the heart because of this influence of the blood vessels in occasioning an irregularity of its action has led to an erroneous and sentimental regard for that organ.

This intricate nervous development suggests the extreme importance of a well-trained organization as a factor toward preventing that broad class of cases which are grouped under the generic title of neurasthenia. In this condition—rather than disease—a similar restlessness and over sensitiveness is present as in profound fatigue. In chronic illness the same symptoms are seen, but when these are complained of without any characteristic signs of

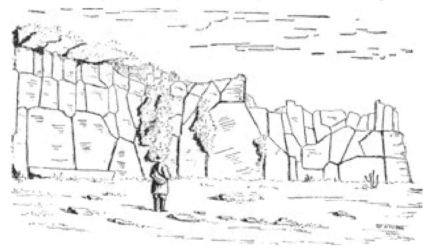

*Cyclopean Wall, Fortressof Sacsahuaman,*
*Back of Cuzco*

disease the indications point to nerve irritability through imperfect elimination of tissue waste. If with this excess of waste materials in the blood there be associated a defective will, then the influence on the sympathetic nerve must be pronounced. Either cause may unbalance the circulation through the arterial system and so disarrange various functions of the body, while a low power of resistance intensifies the mental disability. It is remarkable that these sufferers are at first rarely treated appropriately, but are often impatiently urged to exert will power. While it is undoubtedly true, as so aptly phrased by Shakespeare: "There is no condition, be it good or ill, but thinking makes it so," will power must emanate from a primary store of bodily health.

# Emotions

The greatest factor, however, must be derived through the guidance of the emotions, particularly during the formative period of development. An early education of the will should form a basis for mental control. In this will be found a prominent factor in the production of future happiness, as well as a means of support in many a physical ailment, and even a source of contentment in hopeless disease. But as has already been indicated, the greatest benefit can only result from a healthful working of the entire organism. That there shall be a sound mind in a sound body is an old adage, and recently the great universities have appreciated this sufficiently to officially recognize physical training as an important part of a collegiate education.

Whether the title neurasthenia be scientifically correct for the peculiar train of symptoms which go to make up the complainings of the victims of over-nervous irritability, it has served since the classification of some thirty years ago to enable the acute medical examiner to group the particular sufferers from this morbid condition.

*An early education of the will should form a basis for mental control.*

As defined by Dr. Beard, neurasthenia is: "A chronic functional disease of the nervous system, the basis of which is the impoverishment of nervous force; deficiency of reserve, with liability to quick exhaustion, and the necessity for frequent supplies of force. Hence the lack of inhibitory or controlling powers, both physical and mental, the feebleness and instability of nerve action, and the excessive sensitiveness and irritability, local and general, and the vast variety of symptoms, direct and reflex."

The condition may be summed up as one of nerveless-ness, or a weakness of irritability akin to the symptoms, which indicate profound tire. A host of modern physiolo-gists regard fatigue as due to some poison in the blood. If we accept this theory founded upon chemical facts, which may be clearly demonstrated by experiment, there is ample means for explaining the multiplicity of nervous symp-toms as resulting from this cause alone. Waste matters in the circulation by clogging the capillaries prevent the venous blood from being appropriately purified. The nerve centers do not receive suitable stimulus for repair, and the increased irritability occasions an excessive waste, which still further impedes the circulation. Functional changes must necessarily result in the heart, kidneys, liver and the brain from this continued irritation.

# Nervous Tension

The subjective symptoms of neurasthenia are not so much engendered by a weakness of the nervous system, nor any lack of susceptibility of the nervous protoplasm to respond to irritation, as through excessive irritability, which renders **the** organism over sensitive to normal and healthful stim-ulus. It is a condition, which may be allied to the harp, so strung up as to permit the slightest breath to set its strings in a discordant hum. Often the subjects of this form of trou-ble are found among those who are in the prime of activity, in early adult life, when the various forces for the produc-tion of energy are being vigorously employed.

As it is that part of the body, which is most active at any one period of life—particularly of growth—that is most liable to disease, so during the different epochs of pubes-cence, adolescence, and the early marital life in either sex, the symptoms of neurasthenia may be exhibited. These symptoms are particularly manifest when there has been at these periods a condition of overstrain, associated with

mal-nutrition. Among all possible causes my experience
has been that the genetic factor, through repeated explosive shocks upon the nervous system, is pre-eminent in
the production of neurasthenic symptoms in those already
overworked or suffering from imperfect nutrition.

Neurotics are prone to excesses as well as to extremes in
any particular line. They are the class to which "habits" cling
and "habit drugs" belong, and the apparent candor of their
sufferings might often lead the sympathetic, unwary listener
astray. In such subjects these habits and excesses should be
regarded rather as symptoms than the underlying cause of
the condition. If this fact were more generally thought upon
we should hear less of those who have been wrecked by
alcohol or opium. Indeed it is a fact that a perfectly healthy
man rarely becomes a morphinist, cannabist, etc., but that
such individuals are without exception neuropathic.

The numerous symptoms, which go to make up the
condition of nervous prostration have only been made
prominent through the push for supremacy, and even for
maintenance, in the various specialisms of life. While the
causes always have existed, modern civilization has greatly
exaggerated them, and the present dwellers in cities are
consequently eminently of the nervous type. The sufferers
are not all from one class, but are numbered among the
high, the low, the rich and the poor, though the symptoms
may be varied in accordance with the cultivation and
environment of the patient. What the poor Andean Indian,
working laboriously for days on scanty food, might regard
as the ban of some "spirit of the mountain" cast upon him
for presuming to invade some hallowed precinct and as a
charm against which he chews the sacred Coca, the used
up subject of protracted social functions considers in a different light. But the symptoms and conditions are similar,
whether occasioned from over-indulgence and overwork,
because of exalted ambition, or from enforced labor associated with hygienic errors.

The title neurasthenia has been made responsible for a multitude of evils, quite as bad as has that of "malaria" or "biliousness." "While the group of subjective symptoms which Beard classed under this head has been expanded to embrace about every condition generated from nervous irritability, it remained for the classic guidance of Charcot to accentuate the importance of a certain few symptoms into what he styled "the stigma of neurasthenia," in an effort to combine these as an exact disease.

It is very different whether we consider this classic form or the commonly accepted type. On the one hand there may be mere nervous irritability, while on the other this is accentuated until it approaches the border line of psychical aberration. The more grave condition has been traced from a neurotic heredity or degeneracy, while the simpler application is made to embrace all forms of mental worry, from a mere nervous headache to some pronounced *phobia,* or dread. The two types, however, often intermingle on the threshold of some severe nervous affection, with hypochondriacal, epileptic or paralytic symptoms, or even insanity.

The popular idea of nervous debility held by the laity as well as by the general practitioner in medicine is not the serious disorder of the alienist any more nearly than is a "fit of the blues"—which, since the days of Burton's *Anatomy of Melancholy,* has been attributed to "biliousness"—is true melancholia. The two terms are used by the unknowing or the unthinking ones as interchangeable, the one being a simple temporary mental despondency, which may arise from any one of many causes, while the more serious ailment manifests this condition profoundly and characteristically all the time.

Charcot claimed that neurasthenia was entitled to a definite place in mental pathology, because the disease as witnessed by him maintains its identity under varying circumstances of origin. He believed the condition to be essentially distinct from hysteria, although it might be associated with that disease, and so present a complex hystero-neurasthenia combination which was also described by Beard. That is, the patient may exhibit only neurasthenic symptoms, or united with these the symptoms may be of positive hysteria.

# Morbid Fears

Levillain has, with many other authors, described two varieties of neurasthenia—that from heredity and the acquired. The two forms differ not only in their progress, but in their response to treatment. Among the peculiar train of symptoms commonly seen in this disorder are curious feelings of morbid fear or dread experienced by its subjects. This is similar to the hallucinations which the Germans term *"zwangsvorstellungen"* and *"zwangshandlungen,"* and which others have given a long list of terrible names. *Agoraphobia* is a dread of open spaces, *anthropophobia* is a fear of society, the antithesis of which is *monophobia*—the fear of being alone. Then there is *pantophobia,* a fear of everything, and a culmination which must be the last straw—*phobophobia,* a fear of being afraid. The French term this condition *"peurs maladies." "Folie de doute"* is the name given by Le Grande du Saulle to a condition of chronic uncertainty when there is a morbid doubt about everything.

Hereditary neurasthenia, it is asserted, may develop in those whose parent: were distinctly nervous, even though the usual determining cause may not be present. Among predisposing causes, over-excitation including all forms of overstrain, whether sudden or gradual, is predominant, while the condition is not markedly influenced by alcohol or narcotics. The essential symptoms which Charcot described as the stigmata of the disease are: (1) Headache of a special kind; (2) Digestive troubles; (3) Incapacity for work; (4) Loss or diminution of sexual desire; (5) Muscular lassitude, marked by easily induced fatigue, and painful stiffness; (6) Spinal pain; (7) Insomnia; (8) Hypochondriacal views of life.

Other symptoms which may appear are vertigo, cardialgia simulating angina pectoris, palpitation of the heart, feelings of faintness, and irritable pulse; but these may not be constant. The muscle weakness, with an indescribable irritability expressive of fatigue, Charcot considered so prominent a symptom that he reserved for it the term *"amyosthenia."* The headache is of a peculiar character, suggestive of a weight or constriction over the back of the head or vertex, and sometimes over the whole cranium,

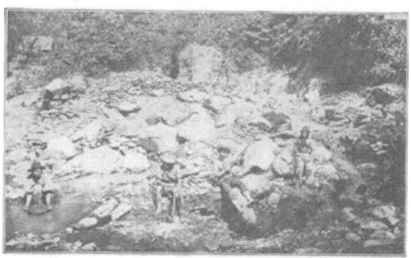

*Indians washing gold from Adrean stream*

described as the "neurasthenic helmet." In some cases this sense of pressure may be hemi-cranial. The insomnia, or troubled sleep, so annoying in pronounced cases, is a very important symptom. The backache may be limited to the sacral region, or to the neck, or may at times be in the coccyx, and is commonly aggravated by pressure. The digestive symptoms are of a general nervous type. With these there is incapacity for mental work, and particularly a lack of concentration of thought.

From the classic grouping it will be seen that it is often difficult to draw the line between actual organic nerve
trouble and neurasthenia. Perhaps the usual type, as seen
by the general practitioner, presents a nerve depression—
an inability of the organism to speedily repair itself after
some call for unusual strain, while the two most prominent
factors of this condition are sleeplessness and mal-assim-
ilation. Under such influences it is easy to understand
that the symptoms presented may be manifest as cerebral,
spinal, genital, chlorotic, vascular, cardiac, or gastric, while
there may be an especial indication pointing toward the
liver. It is quite plausible, as Boix has shown, to have a
"nervous dyshepatia" as well as a nervous dyspepsia, due
to defective innervation.

*Other symptoms which may appear are vertigo, cardialgia simulating angina pectoris, palpitation of the heart, feelings of faintness, and irritable pulse; but these may not be constant.*

It should be understood that the vast array of symptoms which go to make up the condition known as neurasthenia are largely those of reflex irritation, an irritation which may arise from any part of the organism and be transmitted through the sympathetic, and acting chiefly upon the blood vessels through the vaso-motor nerves. It is because of this reflex nature of the symptoms that the condition is often confounded with other diseases, and the sufferer may go the round of the various specialists, and receive "local treatment" for conditions which are erroneously considered to be the chief cause of trouble. What the oculist regards as occasioned from eye strain the rhinologist may look for in the nose. If the patient be a woman, the gynaecologist locates the concentration of troubles in predominant functions. On the other hand, the genito-urinary expert has predetermined that in any nervous man the seat of ills is the prostate gland. It is, therefore, a very common occurrence to find that patients who are nervously irritable have become in themselves multiple specialists. Through constantly going the rounds in search of relief they become familiar with various local conditions, which may give rise to similar symptoms to those they suffer.

These subjects, as a class, are acute and quick; they belong to the clever people, and they are either all elation and prone to overdo or way down "in the blues." It is not surprising then that they soon become familiar with the various remedial efforts toward relieving their symptoms. They not only know in advance what their medical advisers may suggest, but are often prepared to offer a long series of protests against each particular effort toward aiding them to recover from their deplorable condition. If to such a patient, complaining of insomnia, the physician suggests sulphonal—that drug keeps them awake. Then ensues a hasty enumeration of the several hypnotics they have employed, while they recount wherein each had proved in their case an utter failure.

If the symptoms complained of are pronouncedly about the head, they know all about refraction, astigmatism, and the cutting of eye muscles, or they have had their turbinated bodies taken out, or hypertrophied tissue removed from nose or throat, their ears inflated, or they have inhaled and been sprayed to an alarming extent. If by chance the stomach but manifests a twinge of protest, then that poor organ has been dieted and washed, both *gavage* and *lavage*— *ad nauseam*. Thus these patients are commonly treated through all the operative procedures until it is no wonder they should finally become nervous wrecks, ultimately going about from one resort to another, unable to find relief, unable even to find what they deem a competent trained nurse to cater to their imaginings, while a kindly disposed helpmate dances attendance upon their peevish whims.

# Irritable Imaginings

Frequently these cases are subjects of plethoric prosperity, who, if not constitutionally weak, have had no education in self-control. They have spoiled themselves by fretting, and are being more rapidly ruined by petting; the very kindness and consideration that is bestowed upon them at home only adds fuel to their weakness. Often an entire change of environment affords the best condition for the treatment of such cases, such as the rest cure of Weir Mitchell, or one of the German watering establishments, where the regimen is rigid and exact. They must be coerced into recovery or else they will go through the balance of life a nuisance alike to themselves as well as to those who would wish to be their friends. Examples of this condition are legion, and the complainings are as multiple and varied as the ideas of man.

There are instances of self-control when sufferings are held in check while continuing at work. Some of the ablest men in the world's history have been those of weak nervous organization. "Wise judges are we of each other," says Bulwer. Often those whom we look upon as of indomitable will may suffer keenly from some seemingly trivial nervous symptom. A few years ago a prominent justice, who though outwardly was the very picture of health, assured me he suffered more keenly than the abject criminals brought before him, and was literally a coward from nervous dread. He came a long distance for consultation. Possibly it was a satisfaction to get out of his immediate environment and relate his sufferings to one who could listen patiently with a wish to guide him understandingly. Being a popular politician, he was often called upon to make speeches at the most inopportune times—for him, and he seriously proposed to give up a life position because he felt he could not stand the nervous strain.

This is but one example of many similar cases occurring among professional men, with mental faculties constantly at full tension. Whenever there is a lull in their work their thoughts revert to themselves, and the symptoms of an over

*Often those whom we look upon as of indomitable will may suffer keenly from some seemingly trivial nervous symptom.*

tired nervous organism are magnified into some serious physical ailment. These are the cases that maintain the advertising quacks. They wish to be treated confidentially because they would not have their friends know for the world that they are ailing in any particular. They, who are seemingly so strong, would feel humiliated to recount a tale of personal weakness even to a medical man. It can readily be appreciated how necessary it is that a physician shall listen attentively to the story these patients tell, and advise with them openly and candidly as to the plan of treatment, which primarily must consist in some better means of living rather than a dependence upon medication alone. An interchange of confidence between patient and physician, while always advisable, is more necessary in these particular cases than in any other in the entire field of practice of medicine.

There must be faith, and in this much I am an advocate of the faith cure. Indeed, faith is necessary in every walk of life. A chimney may blow off the roof, one may fall on a slippery pavement, a horse may run away, a bridge might fall, a boat might sink, and a hundred and one possibilities might occur to the nervously imaginative. Fear often becomes so exaggerated in the minds of these weak patients that they finally become too timid to attempt anything serious. Such a subject must be assured why and how he is to get well. I once had a patient who would be excited to an indescribable dread if, when walking in the street, he met a truck having any part of the load projecting, such as a chair leg or plank. To avoid it he felt compelled by some uncontrollable influence to turn off into a side street. In another case—a young man, could never go into the society of women, and actually avoided meeting them as much as possible in the street because of an expressed fear that he "must punch them."

These were cases of simple neurasthenia, which appropriate hygienic measures, combined with the administration of Coca—a remedy, which the homoeopaths have long associated as a specific in cases of timidity and bashfulness—completely cured.

The numerous examples which Kraft-Ebing relates of the "Jack the Ripper" order belong to this same class. The complainings of these patients should not be treated flippantly, for the subjects are earnest in their endeavor to find relief from a form of suffering which, while not actually painful, is profoundly humiliating and mentally agonizing. It can be well understood how readily such cases might adopt a drug habit in an unguided effort to find some means of relief.

# Unburdening

There is a tendency in the human mind, which is overweighted to seek support in unburdening a portion of trouble by recounting mental sufferings, whether of illness or not, to another. The celebrated actor, Mr. Frank Drew, related to me a curious example illustrating this, which occurred to him on a recent visit to England. He was dining alone in a restaurant, when a gentleman approached with the remark: "I trust you will not mind if I take a seat at your table V "Not at all," replied the actor; "I shall enjoy company." The two fell into a casual chat, which was resolved into the stranger telling a long and intricate story regarding a purely personal matter, of no interest to an

outsider, yet which was patiently listened to without inter-
ruption to the end.   Then, as though having unbosomed
himself of a weight of woe, he arose, saying:

"You will excuse my having troubled you with this
story, but really it has been a great source of comfort to me
to have found some one to whom I could tell it. Knowing
that we are absolute strangers, and shall never meet again,
I have not hesitated to talk freely to you." On the assurance
of a hearty sympathy, and that the secret should remain
inviolate, they parted, neither expecting to ever see the
other. But it so chanced, in the littleness of this world, that
the following night brought them together again at a dinner party, where they were introduced under embarrassing
recollections.

Not long since, a physician told me of an incident bearing upon this same tendency, which had occurred to him.
One day at the close of his office hours he was preparing
to leave for some outside work, when a lady was ushered
into the consulting room, and instead of relating any physical ailment, entered into a long story of family history,
which was listened to attentively, in expectation that it was
to lead up to the real cause of her visit.

After this story was completed, the relator asked what
she was indebted for the consultation, to which the physician, conscious of his hurry and delay, said in a perfuncto-
ry way: "Five dollars." "Five dollars! Why, I should think
that was altogether too little for having taken up so much
of your time." "Well, then, I will say ten dollars," said the
doctor, treating the whole matter very much as a joke. But
the sincerity was shown by the willingness with which
the fee was extended with the query: "When shall I come
again?" "Say in two weeks," said the consultant smilingly.
"Two weeks! Hadn't I better see you in one week?" "Very
well, make it one week."

And so for several weeks in succession this patient returned and continued to revert to this same story, each time leaving well satisfied after having deposited the customary ten-dollar fee. A case of insanity! Oh, no, merely an over troubled mind which, without apparent physical ailing, had sought relief of mental worries from a physician, who undoubtedly prevented more serious trouble and effected a cure simply through being a good listener. While such instances are not rare in the routine of any practitioner, they seem almost incredible.

# The Mind

I was recently talking with a leading laryngologist, whose practice is in Philadelphia, upon this same line of thought, when he related an anecdote, which had occurred in his own practice. He had gone to Paris for a short visit and had left instructions that his assistant would continue his practice. One day he was visited at his hotel in Paris by one of his Philadelphia patients, who, entering in the most

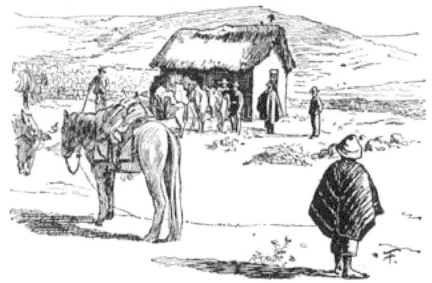

*Andean Tambo at Altitude of 13,500 feet.*

casual way, said: "Doctor, I have a little trouble with my throat I would like to have you look at to-day." The physician, being really surprised to see his patient thus unexpectedly so far

*The mind may excite or depress the various nerve centres, and through these occasion functional changes in muscles or nerves.*

from home, asked him how long he had been in Paris and how long he proposed to remain, and was the more astonished at the reply: "Oh, I just ran over to have my throat treated, and shall take the steamer back tomorrow."

These examples, while in a measure indicating the small-ness of the world, illustrate the fact that patients recognize and require the personal factor in the treatment of their troubles. An element of confidence is established, not necessarily in consequence of any superior preliminary qualifications on the part of the medical man, but because perhaps he has applied his knowledge understandingly.

Dr. Tuke has written scientifically and very entertainingly regarding the subtle relations existing between mind and body—a subject which surely has a very important bearing upon the entire range of functional nervous troubles. The mind has an extraordinary influence, even in health, in causing disorders of imagination, sensation and also of organic functions. An outgrowth from this—a going off as it were on a tangent—leads to various beliefs in phenomena of a superstitious nature and forms a fertile field for the growth of unfortunate methods of treatment; unfortunate because disappointment must follow after the loss of valuable time in experimenting. In this connection I recall a remark made at an alumni dinner by the late Dr. John Hall in speaking of the so-called Christian science: "There is no Christianity in it, and it is not at all scientific."

It is a well-known fact to the physiologist that the mind may excite or depress the various nerve centres, and through these occasion functional changes in muscles or

nerves. I hope it has been conclusively shown that this is
the underlying factor occasioning many of the numerous
subjective symptoms among that immense class known
as neurasthenics. When the famous Dr. John Hunter's
attention was drawn to the phenomenon of animal magnetism—which was exciting the scientific world more than a
century ago, he recognized the possible influence of expec-
tancy upon the imagination, and in his lectures said: "I am
confident that I can fix my attention to any part until I have
a sensation in that part." It is because this possibility of the
influence of the will is overlooked that greater success is
not more commonly met with in the treatment of functional nerve troubles. Mr. Braid emphasized this fact when he
said: "The oftener patients are hypnotized from association
of ideas and habit, the more susceptible they become, and
in this way they are liable to be affected entirely through
the imagination. Thus, if they consider or imagine there is
something doing, although they do not see it, from which
they are to be affected, they will become affected; but, on
the contrary, the most expert hypnotist in the world may
exert all his endeavors in vain if the party does not expect
it, and mentally and bodily comply, and thus yield to it." A
trite application of this thought is the example of the patient who felt "better" as soon as the clinical thermometer
had been placed under his tongue.

## Specifics Infrequent

In the answers received to my inquiry in this research
regarding therapeutic application, fully one-half of those
who went at all into detail advocated the use of Coca for
cases of neurasthenia, and for the various symptoms of
nerve and muscle depression grouped under that title.
The whole train of ills resulting from debility, exhaustion,
overwork, or overstrain of nerve or mind, recalls the early
designation given to the classification of this long group

of symptoms by some of the European physicians as "the American disease," the derangement of an overworked and over hurrying people. The general advocacy of Coca for this condition indicates that the causes which tend to produce such derangement are not only important problems to the general practitioner throughout our country, but must be predominant factors wherever there is an impulse to supremacy. It makes little difference under just what name the symptoms may be treated so long as the patient shall be relieved of suffering.

There is a general idea in the minds of the laity, which, unhappily, is also shared by some physicians, that to name a disease is far more important than its treatment. I well recall, when attending lectures upon medicine, how eager the first year students were to make notes of the various remedies, which each lecturer might advocate for different conditions. It is a difficult task to fill such a therapeutic notebook, but far more difficult to find an appropriate application for the prescriptions suggested. Diseases are of necessity broadly taught in types, and treatment is wholly a result of judgment on the part of the individual practitioner. When a physician has advanced far enough in his struggles in medicine to realize how few specifics there are, he surely broadens himself by cutting loose from the narrow channels of thought he had originally traced in his early student days.

Dr. E. G. Janeway, in a paper before the New York Academy of Medicine, refers to this tendency to treat the name of a disease rather than the condition in the following anecdote:

"Shortly after my entrance into the profession, a fellow interne at the hospital was stricken with a fever, the supposed cause of which was found in the condition of his urine, which contained blood, albumen and casts, and the name of his malady was at this time nephritis. He was given podophyllin to keep his bowels relaxed, and was made

to take a hot bath each day. At the expiration of ten days
of this treatment, an examination showed an eruption. The
name of the disease was changed to typhus fever; the ca-
thartics were discontinued, and in their stead whiskey was
ordered. No marked change was noted in his condition to
call for the change in the treatment; it was simply dependent upon the mental conception of the requirements of
typhus fever then in vogue."

Probably the majority of the laity regard therapy from
the standpoint of specifics. If a proper diagnosis has been
made, the medicine for that particular disease should be
readily forthcoming. If a given prescription does not afford
the relief as speedily as anticipated, the thought is suggested that possibly an error has been made in diagnosis,
and—particularly in the larger cities, this leads to a "going
the rounds" from one physician to another in search of
one who will know "the right medicine." Then again the
ill commonly want a remedy which they can continue for
some particular disease, rather than for any immediate
condition. This unfortunate state of affairs is largely the
fault of the physician in not educating his patients.

While summering in a small country town in the
western part of *New* York State, a hearty Irishman, a farm-
er, called at my office and asked for: "A somethin' for a
kauld," emphasizing his necessity by a gurgling cough that
seemed to rattle from his boots up. On my asking him to
step into the consulting room that I might see just what his
condition was by an examination, he replied in astonish-
ment:

*If a proper diagnosis has been
made, the medicine for that
particular disease should be
readily forthcoming. If a given
prescription does not afford the
relief as speedily*

"Examined, is
it! Sure I've lived
here for the last
twenty-five years,
and never yet was
examined for a kaff

or a kauld!" And he very indignantly left my office to seek some one who would supply him with the needful mixture, for it had been the custom of his usual consultant to give a mixture which might delight the heart of a veterinarian, with some such assurance as he patted a bottle of prodigious size, as: "What ye don't take now will do agen."

If the practice of medicine includes instructing the community as to the limitations of physic, and the necessity for appropriate methods of living, as well as writing prescriptions or dispensing medicines, it would seem that a physician should take pride in teaching his individual patients. It is only by some such method, that in the process of time people will become educated sufficiently to value a conscientious opinion that there is absolutely no trouble and no need for treatment, as of greater monetary worth than a piece of paper ordering something to take to assure a fee.

## Necessity for Guidance

Again, I would impress that in no condition that the physician is called upon to treat is it more necessary to instruct the patient and endeavor to awaken a personal interest and inspire confidence than in the treatment of neurasthenia. These cases, as a class, are so prone to try all sorts of remedies, that they lapse into a condition where it seems as though remedial measures were almost of no avail. Any physician who tries to cure such a patient by the simple administration of medicine alone, or by any one unaided method of local treatment, will find that he has not only a very serious, but hopeless, time-consuming task to perform. Personally I have run the gamut of—I might say, about all methods that have been advocated, and have learned by repeated disappointment how difficult it is to employ one plan. Each case must be studied and treated independently.

From being an early admirer of Dr. Beard's work, I undertook to follow his procedures, not only in medication but in topical treatment. At one time I used electricity very largely and employed the static machine with considerable advantage in some cases. In view of our present knowledge, I hardly believe it will be presumed that this machine simply "strikes awe to the patient," nor that "they see the wheels go round and feel better." With a desire to know more profoundly the rationale for success in this direction, I sought to learn from the manufacturer of my machine— who had also made the instrument used by Dr. Beard, in just what manner he applied it.

I was assured that the handles of his electrodes were made large and long, yet, in spite of this, were frequently being broken. When a suitable case presented, after describing the proposed method of treatment, the patient was asked whether he wished to be cured immediately, or within a space of several months. As may be readily inferred, the majority of patients wished to be cured at once, and so treatment was commenced by a vigorous application of the electrode down the spine, in a manner which combined static sparks with massage in such vigorous blows as to account for the frequent breakage of handles. After this electric attack, the patient was usually quite resigned to accept treatment less severe, "even if it takes more time, doctor."

Here, then, was something of the personal not to be found in this author's works. A mild application of static electricity—that delightful aura—the gentle breeze of ozone which may be wafted from the wooden ball electrode is quite different from the more "magnetic method" described. And it was the method—the force perhaps, the personal magnetism at any rate which rendered the treatment successful.

Neurasthenia is a combination of many symptoms of very different nature; realizing this it is desirable to learn

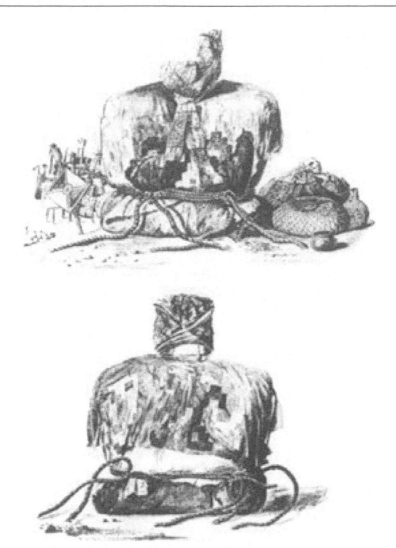

**Peruvian False Head Mummy Packs**

just what these symptoms may be, and whether they are pronouncedly mental or physical. An effort should be made, too, to learn something about the patient, as well as about the cause of complaint—about his work, ambition, hobbies and pleasures. Often these cases necessitate a gradual reparation of many functions before complete cure is to be hoped for, and this will necessitate time. Indeed, time alone with a case under appropriate guidance will work wonders. I usually advocate increasing the activity of the skin by a daily cold sponge bath, taken on rising. Patients quite commonly object to this—they "cannot stand the shock." But it is this very shock that is desirable when indicated. Judiciously used, the physician will find water one of the most useful measures in neurasthenic cases. Indeed, Avithout being an advocate of any "pathy," I believe our friends, the hydrctpaths, certainly deserve much credit for popularizing so simple a remedy. I commonly advise, where there is any trouble with the digestive functions, the drinking of hot water after the method recommended by Dr. Salisbury and so ably advocated by Dr. Ephraim Cutter.

A glassful of water, as hot as can be borne, should be slowly sipped while dressing. Where there is constipation the addition to this of a teaspoonful of Merck's dried sulphate of soda will bring the effects of the best of bitter waters of the German spas home. As to the action of this hot water drinking, I think it cannot be better explained than by repeating a conversation between two clergymen overheard while rummaging through the literary treasures of a book shop. One gentleman was extolling to the other, who was very deaf, the efficacy of drinking a glass of hot water before breakfast—not for deafness, however. To the subdued inquiry from the deaf gentleman as to how it worked, the other shouted: "Sort of washes out the insides," and perhaps this is as much as any of the advocates of this measure can say. It assists in dissolving and washing out the mucus from the stomach, and so prepares that organ for food after the prolonged stage of inactivity of the night.

# Personal Equation

A careful inquiry into the dietary of the patient and a proper regulation of that is always absolutely essential. Without any pet hobbies in this particular, I have often kepi, patients on an exclusive milk diet for months at a time, or again upon a diet of beef and hot water, at times associating with this a liberal supply of grapes. But fruit simply because it is fruit is a delusion as great as the brown bread of Dr. Graham—both should be taken guardedly and advisedly. I believe, with the late Dr. Fothergill, that usually sufferers from nervous troubles do not like fats, while at times they are great lovers of sweets, which by fermentation give an added discomfort. Physiology teaches us that the constituents of nerve cells are chiefly built up from fatty substances, and as the nerves will take from the other tissues it is very reasonable to understand that nervousness and mal-nutrition commonly go together.

Among these subjects the use of milk proves beneficial, because of the contained cream, which is the most easily digested of all fat. And when they will not, or imagine they cannot, drink milk, care should be taken that they shall be instructed how to use it. A patient confined to bed may put on flesh on an exclusive diet of two quarts of milk a day, but one that is up and about, engaged in mental or muscular labor, will require more than this amount.

Dr. Weir Mitchell was an early advocate of absolute rest, enforced feeding, and passive exercise in these nervous cases, which is unquestionably the highest ideal treatment in certain forms of neurasthenia. But where the patient is not ill enough to be put to bed, or will not consent to undertake this ordeal, then the physician must endeavor as nearly as possible to imitate this method by regulating the diet, enforced feeding and massage. In the way of medication and as an adjunct to the food I know of no better remedy than Coca, preferably the original wine of Coca prepared by Mariani. In this the properties of Coca are appropriately preserved by some special method of manufacture, while the mild wine adds a temporary stimulation, which is enhanced by the more permanent influence of the Coca.

# Benefits of Coca

Insomnia is very often an early, persistent and troublesome symptom to be combated. An exhaustion of the brain cells must be repaired just as are the cells of any of the other tissues, through rest and a healthful blood supply. Sleep is the natural rest for the brain, and without this sweet restorer there can be no recuperation from any nervous derangement. I disparage the use of the usual hypnotics and very rarely have recourse to them, except in an emergency—certainly not regularly in any one case.

Yet our patients must sleep, and to establish the habit is going a long way toward ultimate cure. Coca, through its property of clearing the circulation, removes a source of irritation, and may ordinarily be relied upon to induce sleep. When more urgent measures are required the most magical benefit often follows the application of "wet pack." With a case of mania to treat, and with but one remedial measure to employ, I should rely by preference upon the wet pack. Admitting that at first it seems an almost suicidal undertaking to the patient and an alarming procedure to the patient's immediate family, who are anxiously looking on to see fair play, the result is all that could be hoped for. And it is for results that the physician's advice is asked.

To prepare a wet pack the bed is covered with a rubber sheet, and on this a blanket upon which is spread a sheet wrung out of cold water, say at 50° or 00° F. The patient is put naked on this wet sheet, which is quickly wrapped about and tucked in between the legs and arms, so that each limb and the trunk shall be separately enfolded. The underlying blanket is then wrapped about the wet sheet, a hot water bottle is put to the feet, and a cold towel applied to the head. In this condition the subject is permitted to remain from twenty minutes to one or two hours, according to indications. After the first annoyance of seeming imprisonment from the bindings the patient will not mind it any more than does an Indian papoose its wrappings, for pleasant sleep soon follows, or in any case there is a soothed and quieted condition. When the pack is taken off the subject is rubbed dry and tucked up snugly in a dry bed, quite prepared to enjoy a night's restful slumber.

There can be no greater mistake than to continue the use of bromides to allay nervous troubles without some other means added for strengthening the tissues. The bromides, as well as allaying peripheral irritation, always occasion marked depression. It was long since pointed out that Coca equalizes the various forces which constitute energy. A host of observers have remarked that Coca possesses the tranquilizing qualities of the bromides without the depressing effect, and when it is considered necessary to give these salts this depression may be counteracted by Coca, which even dissipates the after effects of chloral, opium and alcohol.

*Sleep is the natural rest for the brain, and without this sweet restorer there can be no recuperation from any nervous derangement.*

In the very nature of things, women are more commonly the sufferers from neurasthenia than are men, because as a rule women are less self-dependent. Formerly such a condition was termed hysteria, because it was supposedly only a disease of women, but since the group of symptoms, which go to make up this condition have been more closely studied, they have been found quite as prevalent among men. It is only another instance of calling things by the wrong name. One who is diffident in society is often called nervous; a trembling old man is nervous; the timid child is nervous; the subject with a weak heart is nervous, as also is very probably the one whose stomach is distended with gas. We are apt to approach matters wrongly; as a result benefits are often lost. Drunkenness, for instance, has occasioned a fearful battle against alcohol, and millions of dollars had been

spent to prove that alcohol caused people to be hopeless
drunkards and wrecks, before it was learned that drunkenness may simply be a manifestation of a diseased nervous
system, while alcohol is really a food often of timely benefit
when rightly used.

Apropos of this thought, there comes to mind the
instance of a recent interview of a professor in one of our
leading colleges who, being interrogated as to his views
regarding the researches of Professor Atwater of Wesleyan
University on "The Nutritive Value of Alcohol," replied
to the query whether he would class alcohol as a food: "If
asked such a question by one of the laity I would reply no,
but if asked by a scientist I must say yes." Unfortunately
there is a tendency in some minds to jump at conclusions,
and to this class the suggestion of food value seems to im-
ply something which can take the place of beefsteak, while
the facts of physiology clearly indicate the definition which
I have formulated: A food is any substance taken into the
body which maintains integrity of the tissues and creates
the energy we term life. But this matter is more fully dis-
cussed in the chapter on dietetics.

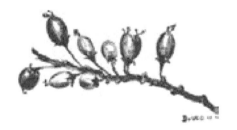

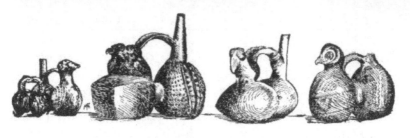

## Chapter 8

# Physiological Action of Coca

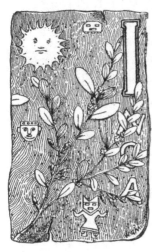

N the study of any scientific problem
the tales and traditions which associate
it with an early race are always full of
interest, for not infrequently there are
hidden among simple and even homely usages suggestive hints. Influences
which among a primitive people were
regarded with superstitious awe, as
of supposed miraculous origin, have
often been developed by knowledge
into important means. Many of the
most useful inventions have thus been
interpreted through the light of science.
The amusing trifles of childhood's hour r ave become the
absorbing powers of the present. Civilization has advanced
by the adaption of primitive means. The history of applied
science has shown this, and is paralleled in the art of medicine, which, while perhaps of slower growth, has evolved
from primeval methods at first regarded as trivial and
empirical, transformations of positive benefit.

If the history of any remedy be traced from its ancient
uses it must be looked for amidst the fables and superstitions of the early people among whom it was associated.
So closely allied has the practice of medicine been with
the mysterious, that many still consider with Bacon, that:

"Witches and impostors have always held a competition with physicians." There has ever been an association of caprice and prejudice in the application of any remedy. This is not merely due to an imperfect knowledge on the part of the physician, but to a false conception among the laity as to the action of medicines or of remedial measures. So when a prosaic real asserts itself over the false ideal, the result has often been an unfortunate scepticism. Science is but the outgrowth of truth, and truth must leave with the advance of time some record of its development.

Quinine came to us through the Incas, who had long been familiar with its uses before the advent of the Count of Chinchon, and although its introduction was clouded in mystery and prejudice, its application as a medicine has been none the less a benefit to millions of people. In the history of Coca, that shrub has been so intimately associated with the everyday customs of the simple people of its native land, that its actual merit remained uninvestigated for ages. For aside from the Spanish prejudice against its employment, the use of Coca was so general that any special effort to seriously study its true qualities seemed unnecessary.

# Evolution from Emiricism

There is a tendency in the human mind to jog along in beaten ruts of old familiar ways without questioning, and so we witness the shallowness of those who have grown up to blindly follow the methods of their predecessors, instead of shaping and adapting the suggestions of earlier times to modern requirements. The natural outgrowth from this spirit is a narrowness of mind, which, while probably asserted to be conservatism, may often be regarded as merely ignorance. For example, one

*There is a tendency in the human mind to jog along in beaten ruts of old familiar ways without questioning.*

may have followed from childhood some certain religion, and yet know absolutely nothing of the doctrines advocated nor any individual reason for accepting them, yet would vigorously resent any innovation upon the customs that were so early grounded, although incapable of offering any plausible support for this narrowness of

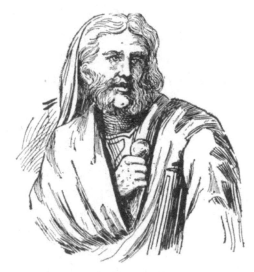

*Claudius Galenus*

view. Such opposition is engendered of weakness, not of strength, it is not built upon true knowledge nor evolved from the logic of unbiased judgment. It is, as my preceptor, the famous anatomist, William Darling, would have said: "False and ridiculous—false because not founded upon fact, and ridiculous because contrary to reason.

Science does not advance a proposition, which cannot be substantiated; hence the purest science is self-evident. It should be as clear and undisputable as Mark Twain would have the proof of Christian Science: "Capable of being read as well backwards as forwards, perpendicularly or sidewise, and bound to always come out the same."

There are relatively few physicians who can logically prove why they employ any certain method, yet these same practitioners would be quick to denounce any medicine used by others in a merely empirical way. The fact that the more familiar remedies are largely empirical has apparently not been recalled. The use of many modern medicines is a simple repetition of methods, which have been continued from the traditions of antiquity. There are probably many

*Linnaeus considered that a medicine differed from a poison not so much in its nature as in its dose.*

who wield potent means who concern themselves little regarding the physiological action of opium or the salicylates, of iodide of potash, of quinine, or mercury, or a host of other drugs in everyday employment.

Even after having accepted a medicine for use the possibilities of its application are not always appreciated. Opium may be a laxative or an astringent, a stimulant or soporific, according to the method of its employment, nor are the whole benefits of the drug to be found in any one of its numerous alkaloids. A similar influence is more prominently manifest in the use of the various varieties of the Coca leaf, or even from the use of Coca of one variety in different preparations. Between such preparations and cocaine—which is commonly regarded as the sole active principle of Coca, the results are still more characteristic.

Linnaeus considered that a medicine differed from a poison not so much in its nature as in its dose, and in this view food, medicine and poison may be considered as intimately allied to each other by indefinable gradations. A common example of this is illustrated in the use of certain condiments. Thus mustard, which, when applied in a small quantity to the food, gives a zest to the appetite, in a large dose acts as an irritant and provokes vomiting.

# Growth of Physiology

It has been the aim of physiologists to learn the working of the human organism, and to trace through the tissues the influence of remedies in health as well as to understand their modified action in disease. The famous school of Alexandria, which flourished two centuries before Christ,

may be regarded as giving
the first inception to physiology, yet for centuries this
science progressed only
by slow stages. Herophi-
lus and Erasistratus were
permitted to practice vivi-
section upon criminals,
an example which was
followed by Fallopius.
These experimenters did
little more than exam-
ine the gross anatomy of
parts, though Herophilus
is considered to have been

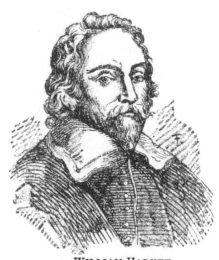

WILLIAM HARVEY.

the first to describe the pulse. But there could be little done
with the intricacies of physiology until minute anatomy
was better understood.

Many of the early philosophers in medicine built theories which were blindly followed by their adherents, just
as has been continued by their successors of the present.
At the beginning of the Christian era Galen, following the
doctrine of *pneuma*—which regarded life as a spirit, taught
that the circulation was a sort of general respiration, the
suction of air filling the vessels "with blood and spirits"
and so causing the wave of pulse. He explained a multitude of qualities and varieties of the pulse, but his theories
were so intermingled with superstition as to command
little respect.

At the period when the Spanish were interested in the
subject of conquests, anatomy and physiology was advancing along with the other sciences. Vesalius, who was
physician to Charles the Fifth of Spain, in his researches
pointed out many errors of Galen, and established the
modern principles of anatomy, while Fal-lopius and Eu-
stachius added the result of their investigations, and Porta

and Kepler, following the earlier hints of Alhazen on re-
fraction, laid a foundation for more perfect knowledge of
the eye. The greatest impetus was given to physiology after
Harvey made known his theory on the circulation of the
blood, which he had built up from the researches of Bacon,
the Spaniard Servetus, the Italian Columbus, the botanist
Csesalpinus, and other famous scholars of the school of
Padua. This advance was supplemented by the work of
Asellius on the lacteals, of Jean Pecquet on the chyle, of
Rlidbeck on the lymph, and by the studies of Malpighi
upon the capillaries and the process of oxygenation of the
blood in the air cells. From this was gradually evolved our
present knowledge regarding the assimilation and transfer-
ence of food into nourishing blood.

Prior to this time it was not known how the tissues were
constructed, nor what were the subtle processes of nourishment—aside from victuals. The science of physiology had
only been dreamed of, and was slowly evolving from a belief in animal spirits and other vague controlling influences
akin to the supernatural. The soul was regarded as the living
force within the body, not only in stimulating the muscles to
contract, but presiding over the secretions. Haller and John
Hunter were the founders of comparative anatomy. The first
was the originator of the doctrine of irritability, which he
showed was not dependent upon the presence of the soul,
and from this originated the experimentation which led to
an understanding of the inherent contractile power of muscle when separated from its nerves.

# Confusion of Stimulants

Cullen, one of the greatest theorists in medicine, displayed
an ingenious system of physiology. He supposed life to consist in an *excitement* of the nervous system, and
especially of the brain, generating a *vital force* which diffused through the animals frame just as electricity pre

vails over nature. In addition to this force he inferred another, which he termed *Vis Medicatrix Naturae*. Through the interaction of both of these there rrrast be maintained a balance to constitute health, while through their unequal activity the problem of disease was to be explained. These teachings were modified by John Brown, who about the commencement of the nineteenth century was private secretary to Dr. Cullen. He taught that life is due to an excitability imparted to every man at his birth and that all disease must belong to either the *sthenic* or *asthenic* diath sis.

The misconception and confusion of the term stimulant originated from the teachings of those ancient philosophers who, in order to offer a physiological explanation for their theory of "vital force," established the supposition of an excitation of tissues from the irritation of stimulus, which they presumed must necessarily be followed by depression. To this has been added a modern confusion through confounding stimulants with intoxicants, which is erroneous in fact. Quickly digested food is a stimulant, a cup of hot water slowly sipped may be a stimulant, and these or *any substance which increases natural action*—which is the true definition of stimulant—will not necessarily be followed by a period of depression corresponding to the previous sense of well being. Nor does a proper stimulant irritate to fretful excitement. The true stimulant simply rouses latent energies, which may be quite capable to work if only suitable impetus be given to promote activity.

One of the most able writers upon this subject has placed quickly digested and nutritious food at the head of stimulants, of which all other means can but be the faint reflex. Under such action, the pulse is given increased firmness without hurry and there is less feeling of fatigue, while a grateful warmth pervades the body, accompanied by a general sense of well being. These indeed are the physiological results of a good meal or may similarly follow from the use of Coca.

These facts have been interpreted by many observers, and although it is not claimed that Coca replaces beefsteak, certainly it may in emergency act as a substitute for a more ample dietary, or may advantageously be used at other times to stimulate the assimilation and conversion of other food. It is the reconstructive action upon the tissues, which forms one great benefit of the wide range of usefulness of Coca.

For more than three centuries the information that had come to the world in regard to Coca had been chiefly of a theoretical nature. The writings of travellers and of missionaries who were located in the sections of South America where Coca was used, had prepared the way for a scientific investigation of its properties as soon as there was a possibility of such work being done with exactitude. After the botanists had classified the plant, and chemists had begun to search for the hidden properties of its traditional action, the researches of the physiologists soon followed.

# Experiments With Coca

In Europe the attention of the medical profession was directed to the action of Coca through a widely circulated

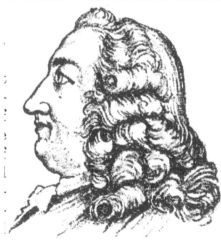

ALBERT HALLER.

paper by Dr. Mantegazza, who experimented upon himself, using the leaves both by chewing and in infusion. His description, while somewhat fanciful and full of imagination, fairly illustrates the physiological action of Coca, provided it is appreciated that observations made by an experimenter upon his own person are necessarily influenced by the temperament of the individual. He found from masticating a drachm of the dried leaves: "An aromatic taste in the mouth, an increased flow of saliva, and a feeling of comfort in the stomach, as though a frugal meal had been eaten with a good appetite." Following a second and a third dose there was a slight burning sensation in the mouth and pharynx with an increased pulse beat, while digestion seemed to be more active.

Through the influence of Coca the entire muscular system is increased in strength with a feeling of agility and an impulse to exertion quite different from the exaltation following alcohol. While from the latter there may be increased activity, it will be of an irregular character, but Coca promotes a gradual augmenting of vigor with a desire to put this newly acquired strength in action. Mantegazza found that the intellectual sphere participates in the general exaltation produced by Coca, ideas flow with ease and regularity, the influence being quite different from that induced by alcohol and resembling in some degree that from small doses of opium. After drinking an infusion of four drachms of leaves he experienced a peculiar feeling as though isolated from the external world, with an irresistible inclination to exertion, which was performed with phenomenal ease, so that though in his normal condition he naturally avoided unnecessary exercise, he was now so agile as to jump upon the writing table, which he did without breaking the lamp or other objects upon it.

Following this period of activity came a state of quietness accompanied by a feeling of intense comfort, consciousness being all the time perfectly clear. The experimenter took as much as eigh-

*Through the influence of Coca the entire muscular system is increased in strength with a feeling of agility and an impulse to exertion quite different from the exaltation following alcohol.*

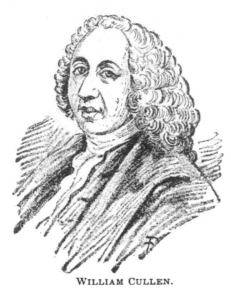

WILLIAM CULLEN.

teen drachms of leaves in one day, which is about the amount ordinarily consumed by the *Serrano* of the Andes. Under this increased dose the pulse was raised to one hundred and thirty-four, and when mental exhilaration was most intense he exclaimed to his colleagues who were watching the result of his investigation: "God is unjust because he has created man incapable to live forever happy."[3] And again: "I prefer a life of ten years with Coca to a life of a million centuries without Coca." Following these experiments, during which he had abstained from any food but Coca for forty hours, he took a short sleep of three hours, from which he woke without any feeling of indisposition.

Dr. Mantegazza announced as a result of the studies made upon himself and verified upon other subjects that Coca, chewed or taken in a weak infusion, has a stimulating effect on the nerves of the stomach and facilitates digestion. That it increases the animal heat, and the frequency of the pulse and respiration. That it excites the nervous system in such a manner that the movements of the muscles are made with greater ease, after which it has a calming effect, while in large doses it may cause cerebral congestion and hallucinations. He asserted that: "The principal property of Coca, which is riot to be found in any other remedy, consists in its exalting effect, calling out the power of the organism without leaving any sign of debility, in which respect Coca is one of the most powerful nervines and analeptics." From these conclusions he advocated the use of Coca in disorders of the alimentary tract, in debility following fevers, in anaemic conditions, in hysteria and hypochondriasis, even when the latter has increased to suicidal intent. He considered that Coca might be used with benefit in certain mental diseases where opium is commonly prescribed, and was convinced of its sedative effect in spinal irritation, idiopathic convulsions and nervous erethism, and suggested its use in the largest doses in cases of hydrophobia and tetanus.

# A Heart Tonic

Some of the assertions of Mantegazza are directly opposed by our present knowledge of the action of Coca, particularly the observations as to its action on the heart and respiration. This is to be accounted for by the pronounced central action he observed, evidently prompted by a belief that the influence of Coca was primarily through the nervous system. It has been developed by more recent research that Coca has a direct action upon the muscular system. The action of Coca upon the heart is precisely as a regulator of that organ. If the heart's action is weak it is strengthened—if it is excessive the over-activity is toned down—if irregular the beat is made uniform. This indicates that Coca is a direct cardiac tonic. **Let** the heart be running riot in a palpitation from over-exertion and a teaspoonful of Mariani The—taken in a small cup of hot water—will speedily bring the heart's action to normal. This unique preparation of Coca is in the form of an agreeable fluid extract, said to represent in one part, two parts of the leaves, and presenting in concentrated form all the qualities of true. Coca. It may be administered plain, or drunk as a tea with cream and sugar; in this latter form it has a taste resembling a rich English breakfast tea.

The especial influence of Coca upon the heart is alone sufficient to establish it as a remedy of phenomenal worth.

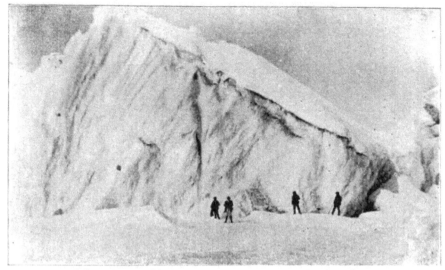

*Glacier of Mt Ananea – at 17,000 feet.*
*Cordillera of Aricoma, Peru*

Lieutenant Gibbs, U. S. N. from a personal experience with Coca in crossing the high passes of the Andes, considered the sustaining action of Coca in high altitudes due wholly to its enabling the heart muscle to perform the extra work then called forth. Similar observations have been made by many travellers who have remarked the influence of Coca upon themselves. Recently, Captain Zalinski, IT. S. A.— who rendered the dynamite gun an effectual instrument of war—has been experimenting upon a concentrated ration suitable for the army. In pursuing his studies under a severe test he submitted himself to the hardships of Andean travel, and through the high altitudes used Coca The and Coca Pate prepared by Mariani, the timely use of which, he assured me, had supported his life through a serious ordeal.

Dr. Beverley Robinson, referring to the efficiency of heart tonics has written: "Among well known cardiac tonics and stimulants for obtaining temporary good effects, at least, I know of no drug quite equal to Coca. Given in the form of wine or fluid extract, it does much, at times, to restore the heart muscle to its former tone." In this connection, Dr. Ephraim Cutter says: "Coca should be more used in heart failure from direct weakness, and in many cases might well replace the conventional digitalis which advances the treatment of heart disease no more than it was forty years ago." Coca is advocated to replace digitalis or to tone up the muscular structure of the heart after use of the latter, either employed alone or alternately with digitalis when that is considered essential!

The effect of Coca upon respiration is analogous to its action on the heart. It acts as a regulator, not increasing respiration, but giving force to the cycle—making inspiration deeper and expiration more complete.

# Introduction of Cocaine

The observations of Mantegazza were followed by Niemann's researches upon cocaine, that the mistaken conception originated that the phenomenal activity of Coca had been discovered in that alkaloid, and subsequent physiological work was almost wholly carried out upon cocaine with the resultant neglect of the parent plant. The reports of many of the earlier experimenters, however, were so contradictory as to give rise to a suspicion whether cocaine had been used at all.

But as the substance employed had been obtained from Coca leaves, and as the investigators were familiar with the methods of physiological research, this variation suggested some probable difference in the quality of cocaine used, which it was presumed was brought about in the process of manufacture. This varying result has since been shown to have been occasioned by a mixture, in various proportions, of the Coca bases contained in the earlier specimens of cocaine, before they had been appreciated as distinct products.

Schroff was one of the first to experiment with the new
alkaloid. He observed that cocaine produces a slight anaesthesia of the tongue, and gives an agreeable sense of lightness of the mind with a condition of cheerfulness and well
being, followed by lassitude and an inclination to sleep.
From augmented doses he remarked giddiness, buzzing in
the ears, dilatation of the pupils, impaired accommodation,
headache, restlessness, and a feeling as though walking
upon air. The heart was first quickened and then retarded. There was no reaction from the motor nerves, and the
respiration was lowered from smaller doses. Demarle, who
experimented about the same time with Coca, remarked
the anaesthesia from chewing the leaves and the dilatation
of the pupils noticed in his own person.

In 1865, Dr. Fauvel, of Paris, used a preparation of Coca
which had been prepared for him by Mariani as a local application, to relieve pain in the larynx, and this treatment was
continued in England by Dr. Morrell Mackenzie and in the
United States by Dr. Louis Elsberg, who had remarked the
beneficial effects of this application in Fauvel's clinic. It seems
remarkable that no general use was made of this anaesthetic
property for nearly a quarter of a century after these early observations until cocaine was adapted by Dr. Carl Koller to the
surgery of the eye. A great many erroneous accounts of this
adaptation have been published, but I am assured this gentleman never wrote nor authorized any writing upon cocaine
except the preliminary paper and his principal paper before
the *Gesellschafl der Arzte* at Vienna, and later his article in the
*Reference Handbook?* but in none of these is given the details
which led to the surgical uses of cocaine.

At the period of his experiments Dr. Koller was
*Sekun-dararzt,* or house surgeon, on the staff of the *k. k.
Allgemeinen Krankenhauses,* the largest hospital of Vienna,
which serves also as a clinic for the medical faculty of the
University. Through his connection with Professor Strieker
he had been interested in experimental physiology and

pathology and had made considerable research in the action of poisons upon the circulation. His investigations upon cocaine were therefore in a similar nature to those with which he was familiar. In August, 1884, Dr. Sigmund Freud and Dr. Joseph Breuer, of the University of Vienna, treated a prominent physiologist for morphinism by the use of

*The discovery was made accidentally when a student had in mistake applied a solution of cocaine to the eye of a friend. Instead of the irritation feared from this carelessness, the property of dilatation and anaesthesia was found.*

cocaine, which had about then been prominently advocated in American literature. Several of the hospital staff were induced to try the effects of the alkaloid upon themselves.

Among these was Dr. Koller, who, from a dose of the salt taken internally, remarked the benumbing action upon the tongue, which had already been recorded by other observers. He had before been looking for a local anaesthetic, and with this in view had experimented with morphine, chloral, the bromides, and a number of other substances, so when he experienced the numbness from cocaine he realized he had found the sought-for anaesthetic, and experimented to determine its utility in ophthalmology.

It has been asserted that this discovery was made accidentally, and the story is related that a student had in mistake applied a solution of cocaine to the eye of a friend, when instead of the irritation feared from this carelessness, the property of dilatation and anaesthesia was found. Dilatation of the pupil had previously been noted from cocaine, but anaesthesia could hardly be observed accidentally, and, indeed, was determined not by local but by physiological experimentation. It had been known that the action of Coca through the circulation contracts the peripheral arteries, also that it dilates the pupil. Tschudi wrote: "After mastication of a great quantity of the Coca the eye seems unable to bear light and there is marked distention of the pupil." An effect which had ako been noted by many other observers.

# Experiments With Cocaine

Koller's experiments were carried out in the laboratory of Professor Strieker upon guinea pigs. It was found that a minute quantity of a solution of hydrochlorate of cocaine dropped in the conjunctival sac, produced such complete local anaesthesia that the cornea could be irritated with needles and electric currents and cauterized with nitrate of silver until it became opalescent. This experiment suggested that anaesthesia was not merely upon the surface but involved the entire thickness of the cornea. After experimenting upon animals the investigator applied cocaine to his own eye and examined the efficiency of the anaesthetic in diseased eyes. A preliminary paper upon the result of this discovery was sent to the annual meeting of the *Deutsche Ophthalmologiche Gesellschaft,* held at Heidelberg Sept. 15-16, 1884, which was read by Dr. Brettauer of Trieste. With this paper was a vial containing a few grammes of cocaine, which was all of the alkaloid that Merck could furnish at that time.

Meantime Roller continued his experiments and asked specialists in other departments to employ the alkaloid in their practice, for though satisfied that he had found a local anaesthetic adapted to the surgery of the eye, he believed that it was also suited to other special uses, a fact soon confirmed by several observers who based their researches upon this original investigation. This, briefly, is the story of the adaptation of this alkaloid of Coca to minor surgery, which is modestly all the merit of "discovery" that is claimed by the one through whom cocaine has been made a boon to suffering humanity, fully as important, and in many cases superior to the great anaesthetics, chloroform and ether.

When a two per cent, solution of cocaine is applied to the eye there is at first a slight irritation, followed by a drying of the secretions. The pupil is dilated and the eye has a staring look, occasioned from a wider opening of the lids. Anaesthesia continues for about ten minutes, followed by a stage of reduced sensibility, slowly passing into the normal condition. Dilatation reaches the highest stage within the first hour, decreases considerably in the second hour, and then soon disappears entirely. The pupil is never at a maximum dilatation; that is, it may always be further dilated with atropine, and still responds to light and convergence.

The dilating power of cocaine combined with atropine is invaluable when used in cases of iritis, the combination counteracting both the muscular spasm and the local congestion. In this condition Koller uses equal parts of a five per cent, solution of hydro-chlorate of cocaine, with a one per cent, solution of sulphate of atropine. After the dilatation following a few applications the solution is used three times a day.

At first it was supposed that local anaesthesia from cocaine was due to anaemia of the minute vessels, but it was found that though anaemia followed an application of the alkaloid the anaesthesia preceded this influence. That the benumbing action was not only local but might be general through the circulation was subsequently shown by the subcutaneous injection of a solution of the salt. Half a grain of hydrochlorate of cocaine so used occasioned a slight general anaesthesia, while repeated injections of small doses caused a general reduction of tactile sensibility, with the sensation as though standing on cushions. This was similar to the floating in the air experience of Mantegazza from large doses of Coca, and is in accord with the observation of Schroff with cocaine. The symptom is due to a lessened power of conduction in the cord.

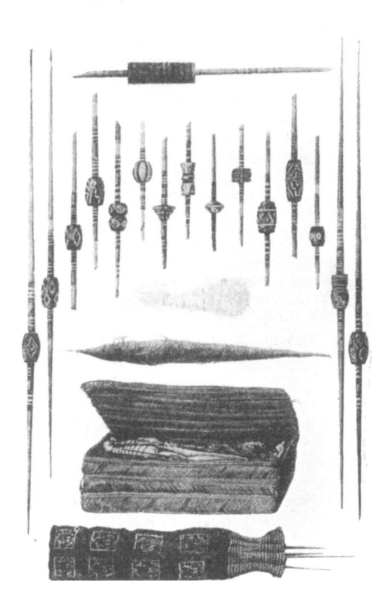

*Incan Spinning Spindles and Work Basket*

From an injection of 0.001 gramme of hydrochlorate of cocaine under the skin of the abdomen of a monkey, not only local but general anaesthesia was produced which lasted for eighteen minutes without loss of consciousness. It has been suggested that absence of tactile sensibility may give rise to the impression in the observer that consciousness in the subject is lost. From the fact that a subcutaneous injection of cocaine at any point eases pain, it has been presumed that the action must be central as well as local. But general anaesthesia has been shown to follow only from very large doses. While diminished sensibility may presumably be induced from a central cause, the fact has been pointed out that lessened conduction in the cord is a more potent factor in diminishing the general sensibility than any narcotic action upon the brain.

# Affinity of Alkaloids

Cocaine has not only the property of exciting the brain, but the special senses may be inhibited by a dose sufficient to paralyze their terminal nerve endings. Thus powdered hydrochlorate of cocaine blown into the nostrils first occasions increase and then total abolition of the sense of smell. Koller observed that an injection of cocaine solution in the orbit occasioned loss of light in an eye he was about to remove.

It has been remarked by physiologists in experimenting with alkaloids that there is a relation between the constitution of the chemical molecule and the physiological action. The introduction of methyl into the molecule of strychnine, brucine and thebaine changes the convulsive action of these substances on the spinal cord to a paralyzing one exerted on the ends of the motor nerves. Probably any of the organic alkaloids in which methyl and ethyl enter would paralyze both muscle and nerve, the latter before the former, the symptoms varying in accordance with the order

*An enormous dose of atropine is required to paralyze the motor nerves, but a very small dose is sufficient to affect the nerves of the heart and other involuntary muscles, and thus we get rapid circulation, dilated pupil and restless delirium.*

in which different parts of the nervous system may be affected.

The activity depends also upon the affinity, which the substance may have for certain tissues which through alteration of function may affect the organism, and this accounts for the difference manifest between a large and a small dose. This is illustrated by atropine and by curare either of which paralyze motor nerves, but while a very large dose of curare is necessary to paralyze the cardiac and vascular nerves a small dose paralyzes the nerves going to the muscles. On the other hand, an enormous dose of atropine is required to paralyze the motor nerves, but a very small dose is sufficient to affect the nerves of the heart and other involuntary muscles, and thus we get rapid circulation, dilated pupil and restless delirium. The influence of these radicals in the Coca bases has already been referred to. The researches of several investigators indicate that cocaine is a protoplasmic poison, first stimulating, then paralyzing the vital functions, but it is possible to regulate this action so that the functions may be either increased or held in check even in minute organisms.

The motion of amoebae in normal salt solution was stopped by a two per cent, solution of cocaine and the movement of spermatozoids and of ciliated cells was checked by stronger solutions. Claude Bernard long since explained that cell metabolism in the lower organisms—in which the contractile protoplasfn fulfills both the function of nerve and of muscle—may be suppressed by chloroform narcosis, the phenomenon being identical with that observed in anaesthesia of animals. In such anaesthesia there is inhibition of cell activity and not necessarily death of cell substance. He has shown by experiment upon plants that while growth and cell division ceases when under the influence of the anaesthetic, vitality is resumed when the plant is again under normal healthful conditions.

This influence follows upon the use of cocaine. The cell life is first stimulated and if the dose is increased there is inhibition, but activity is resumed upon the withdrawal of the drug. Similar results were obtained in my research made in the laboratory of the botanical department of Columbia University. It was found that both Coca and cocaine have a marked stimulating influence upon the lower organisms.

My experiments were made with *infusoria,* yeast, *penicillium* and the aquatic plant *Elodea,* which latter forms a common substance for illustrating in the laboratory the effect of metabolism as represented by the bubbles of oxygen given off under the action of various stimuli. Portions of this plant exposed in test tubes to similar conditions of water, temperature and sunlight exhibited under the influence of Coca a stimulated metabolism as shown by the relative increase of bubbles, from twenty in twenty-eight seconds in the standard, to twenty in seven seconds in the tubes to which small portions of Coca The or solution of cocaine had been added. A similar result was obtained from the increased growth of the yeast plant in a solution of sugar, as indicated by the decomposition of the carbohydrate.

In each of four graduated test tubes there was placed fifteen cubic centimetres of a solution of sugar and yeast. One of these was left normal. To the others there was added respectively one, two and three cubic centimetres of a one per cent, solution of cocaine. The relative activity of metabolism was increased above the standard, twenty-five per cent, fifty per cent, and twenty-five per cent, the latter indicating the excitation limit for these particular organisms had been passed.

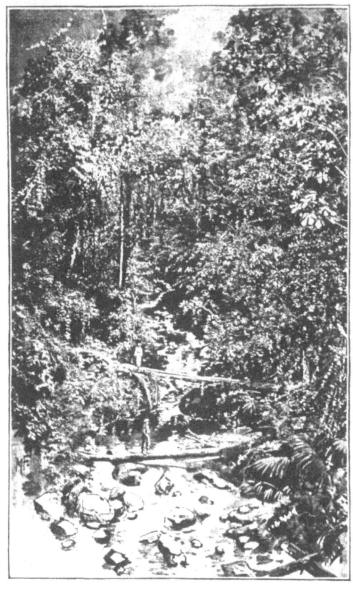

*In the Heart of Montana.*

In studying the growth of *penicillium,* upon which Dr. Curtis was then engaged in making an exhaustive series of experiments upon turgor, I had the privilege of examining specimens prepared by this skilled microscopist of drop cultures growing in a nutrient solution. There was a very marked influence to be seen in the rapidity of growth, which was readily measured under the microscope and compared with similar specimens to which no Coca had been added.

# The Spinal Cord

The influence of cocaine upon sensory nerves may be effected not only by local application but by a direct application to the nerve trunks, and even by an application to the nerve centres in the cortex. In 1885 Dr. Corning experimented with anaestlietization of the spinal cord, and injected thirty minims of a three per cent, solution of hydrochlorate of cocaine between the spinous processes of the lower dorsal vertebrae in a subject suffering from spinal weakness. Sensibility was impaired in the lower limbs and the patellar reflexes were abolished. There was but slight dilatation of the pupils and no incoordination or motor impairment discernible, but the patient experienced dizziness while standing and was mentally exhilarated. Dr. Bier of Kiel has recently suggested a general anaesthesia from cocaine by injecting by means of a Pravaz syringe from three to five cubic centimetres of a one per cent, solution of hydrochlorate of cocaine directly into the vertebral canal. Following the injection complete anaesthesia of the lower limbs took place within eight minutes, gradually mounting as high as the nipple; complete insensibility to pain lasted about forty-five minutes. The serious nature of this procedure is sufficient to condemn the process for general use, in view of less dangerous methods.

It has been suggested that as the local influence of cocaine in moderate doses is chiefly exerted upon sensory nerves, large doses occasion a sensory paralysis which may even extend to the motor branches. It has been shown, however, that the motor terminals are only indirectly paralyzed either through an anaesthetic action upon the skin or from an action upon the muscle through which the nerve passes, and in this way the motor nerves may be affected. A number of observers have found, from experiments upon lower animals, the motor nerves depressed, or a diminution of muscle irritability from cocaine only after very large doses, while others have observed muscular paralysis without previous stimulation. But as alteration of sensibility always precedes the symptom of motor paralysis, the apparent lack of motion may be attributed to the former cause. Thus, Mosso describes having pressed his whole weight on the foot of a dog under the influence of a large dose of cocaine, without causing movement. Other observers have failed to note any direct effect upon muscle from cocaine.

The action of cocaine seems more pronouncedly upon the central nervous system, while the properties of Coca appear to be controlled by its associate alkaloids to affect muscle as well as nerve. The influence of Coca to excite muscle to energy is probably due to a direct chemical action toward the construction of proteid, as well as through the excitation of the hypothetical ferment of the contractile element, as has already been explained in the chapter upon muscle. The pronounced bearing which the associate alkaloids of Coca may exert, to maintain the balance of energy in

*The action of cocaine seems more pronouncedly upon the central nervous system, while the properties of Coca appear to be controlled by its associate alkaloids to affect muscle as well as nerve.*

favor of the leaf above one of its alkaloids, may be appreciated from a consideration of the distinctive physiological action of several of the more important active principles of Coca.

A physiological study of all the Coca products has not been made, but Professor Ralph Stockmann instituted an important research in this direction at the University of Edinburgh. From these experiments, it has been shown that the action of certain of the Coca alkaloids is directly upon muscular tissue; notably among these may be mentioned *ecognine, benzoylecognine, cocamine* and *hygrine*. The influence of *ccgonine* upon the central nervous system is so mild that only large doses occasion slight depression, followed by increase of reflex irritability of the spinal cord which may last for several days. The substance has no ansesthetic properties, and the motor nerves are not specially influenced.

## Muscular Alkaloids

There is, however, a lessening of the irritability of muscles, those having the largest blood supply being most deeply affected. When the drug was pushed to poisonous doses death followed from extension of the rigor mortis to a large number of muscles. The effect of *benzoylecgonine* is directly upon muscle in a manner somewhat similar to caffeine, inasmuch as it provokes a muscular stiffness; this was followed, as late as the third or fourth day, by a slight increase in reflex excitability which upon increase of the drug tended to tetanus. This late manifestation of spinal symptoms is due to the fact that benzoylecgonine has so great an affinity for muscle, that it is imbibed by adjacent muscles so thoroughly that the more distant structures receive at first very little of the drug.

Non-striped muscle is not so much affected, and the heart is less involved. In cats one gramme (15.43 grains), occasioned dilatation of the pupils, great increase of the reflexes, and diarrhoea. From a poisonous dose death followed when a large number of muscles were affected, or after the spinal symptoms had been severe and long continued. The post mortem appearance revealed the remarkable influence of this alkaloid upon muscle by pronounced contractions of the intestines and bladder. *Cocamine,* which is a local anaesthetic, bears a nearer resemblance to cocaine in its action than do the other Coca alkaloids. While it exhibits the effect of a general stimulant its action is so specifically upon muscle that its influence on the spinal cord is masked. Administered to a frog the animal became alert, excited, restless, and leaped in excess of its usual performance. There was an increase of the reflexes, and the signs of nervous and muscular symptoms continued for several days. The pupils, at first dilated, under an excessive dose became extremely small. The condition of the motor nerves and spinal cord was practically the same as in cocaine poisoning, though the motor nerves were more profoundly influenced.

The nervous system was only affected after the alkaloid had left the muscle and entered the circulation. Cocamine, which is more lethal than is cocaine, when given in a small dose to a cat, occasioned excitement, dilatation of the pupils, twitching of the tail, ears, etc., while an increased dose caused muscular and nervous depression, vomiting, diarrhoea and weakness of gait, all of muscular origin. Death followed many hours after administration of a poisonous dose, and resulted either from rigor mortis of the respiratory muscles, or when more rapid from paralysis of the respiratory center. Post mortem there was constriction of the stomach, intestines and bladder so strongly marked as to cause hour-glass contraction. *Hygrine,* injected under the skin of a frog, occasioned depression, weakness in gait and dullness for a day or two, with tendency to starting and tremors. Its probable effect upon muscle was shown after death by hypersemic spots, scattered throughout the muscular structure and serous membranes, where it had been carried by the circulation. Locally, to the experimenter's tongue, hygrine caused burning and tingling, the former soon passing off, but the latter lasting for an hour.

Stockmann, in experiments upon the frog, using Merck's *hydrochlorate of cocaine,* verified, or rather harmonized the accounts of numerous earlier investigators. He found that cocaine in a moderate dose created a slight torpor with depression of both brain and spinal cord, the symptoms being of sensory rather than of motor depression. The pupils were dilated. There was no stage of excitement. Under an increased dose these conditions were all exaggerated, particularly the reflex to sensory impressions, which now resembled those present in a late stage of strychnine poisoning. With excessive doses there was sensory and motor paralysis, and the pupils were contracted to mere slits. The spinal cord seemed to be given an increased excitability, its discharges being rapid, while it appeared less sensitive to stimuli from the skin and was readily exhausted. In rabbits, it was found that the convulsions occurring in cocaine poisoning could be prevented by artificial respiration.

In considering the action of any of the Coca alkaloids on man, it may be well to suggest that possibly one cause of conflicting testimony may have resulted from reporting the influence of the alkaloid upon animals, the effects of which are not always uniform with their action on man. In experiments upon animals those symptoms which follow doses full enough to create some outward sign are alone seen, while the agreeable exaltation such as would be experienced in man from a relatively much smaller dose can not be appreciated. A dose of cocaine which in one of the lower animals would cause depression, would under the controlling influence of a greater cerebral development in

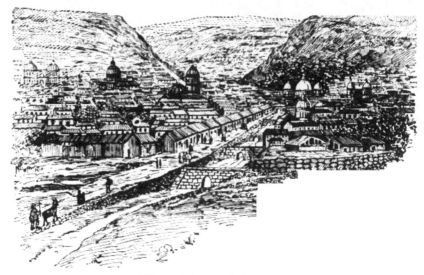

*The City of Cuzco.*

man occasion exhilaration, an effect probably resulting from inhibition of certain of the brain cells, thus inducing slight loss of co-ordination similar to that following a small dose of opium or alcohol. Both alcohol and opium seriously disturb the normal relations of one part of the brain with another, the nerve centers being paralyzed in the inverse order of their development. The primary exhilaration being succeeded by a narcotic action when the inhibitory paralysis permits the emotions full sway. Coca, however, appears to stimulate the brain by an harmonious influence on all the brain cells so the relation of its functions is not deranged.

# Depurative Influence

The action of cocaine has been placed midway between morphine and caffeine. In man the initial effect of Coca is sedative, followed by a rapidly succeeding and long continued stimulation. This may be attributed to the conjoined influence of the associate alkaloids upon the spinal cord and brain, whereby the conducting powers of the spinal cord are more depressed than are the brain centers. In view of these physiological facts it is unscientific to regard strychnine as an equivalent stimulant to Coca or a remedy which may fulfill the same indications, as erroneously suggested by several correspondents. For immediate stimulation Coca is best administered as a wine, the mild exhilaration of the spirit giving place to the sustaining action of Coca without depression. The action of Coca and cocaine, while similar, is different. Each gives a peculiar sense of well being, but cocaine affects the central nervous system more pronouncedly than does Coca, not—as commonly presumed—because it is Coca in a more concentrated form, but because the associate substances present in Coca, which are important in modifying its action, are not present in cocaine. The sustaining influence of Coca has been asserted to be due to its anaesthetic action on the stomach, and to its stimulating effect on brain and nervous system.

But the strength-giving properties of Coca, aside from mild stimulation to the central nervous system, are embodied in its associate alkaloids, which directly bear upon the muscular system, as well as the depurative influence which Coca has upon the blood, freeing it from the products of tissue waste. The quality of Coca we have seen is governed by the variety of the leaf, and its action is influenced by the relative proportion of associate alkaloids present. If these be chiefly cocaine or its homologues the influence is central, while if the predominant alkaloids are coca-mine or benzoyl ecgonine, there will be more pronounced influence on muscle. When the associate bodies are present in such proportion as to maintain a balance between the action upon the nervous system and the conjoined action upon the muscular system, the effect of Coca is one of general invigoration.

*The strength-giving properties of Coca are embodied in its associate alkaloids, which directly bear upon the muscular system,*

It seems curious, when reading of the marvelous properties attributed by so many writers to the influence of Coca leaves, that one familiar with the procedure of the physiological laboratory should have arrived at any such conclusion as that of Dowdeswell, who experimented with Coca upon himself. After a preliminary observation to determine the effect of food and exercise he used Coca "in all forms, solid, liquid, hot and cold, at all hours, from seven o'clock in the morning until one or two o'clock at night, fasting and after eating, in the course of a month probably consuming a pound of leaves without producing any decided effect." It did not affect his pupil nor the state of his skin.

It occasioned neither drowsiness nor sleeplessness, and none of those subjective effects ascribed to it by others. "It occasioned not the slightest excitement, nor even the feeling of buoyancy and exhilaration which is experienced from mountain air or a draught of spring water." His conclusion from this was that Coca was without therapeutic or popular value, and presumed: "The subjective effects asserted may be curious nervous idiosyncrasies." This paper, coming so soon after the publication of a previous series of erroneous conclusions made by Alexander Bennett, created a certain prejudice against Coca.

Theine, caffeine and theobromine having been proved to be allied substances, this experimenter proceeded to show that cocaine belonged to the same group. As a result of his research he determined that "the action of cocaine upon the eye was to *contract* the pupil similar to caffeine," while the latter alkaloid he asserted was a *local* anaesthetic; observations which have never been confirmed by other observers. In view of our present knowledge of the Coca alkaloids, it seems possible that these experiments may have been made with an impure product in which benzoyl-ecgonine was the more prominent base. However, the absolute error of Bennett's conclusions has been handed down as though fact, and his findings have been unfortunately quoted by many writers, and even crept into the authoritative books.

Thus Ziemssen's *Cyclopaedia of the Practice of Medicine,* which is looked upon as a standard by thousands of American physicians, quotes Bennett in saying: "Guaranine and cocaine are nearly, if not quite, identical in their action with theine, caffeine and theobromine." The *National Dispensatory* refers to the use of Coca in Peru as being similar to the use of Chinese tea elsewhere—as a mild stimulant and diaphoretic and an aid to digestion—which are mainly the properties of coffee, chocolate and guarana, and Bennett is quoted to prove that the active constituents of all these products: "Although unlike one another and procured from totally different sources possess in common prominent principles, and are not only almost identical in chemical composition, but also appear similar in physiological action." These statements, which are diametrically opposed to the present accepted facts concerning Coca, are not merely a variance of opinion among different observers, but are the careless continuance of early errors, and suggest the long dormant stage in which Coca has remained, and has consequently been falsely represented and taught through sources presumably authentic.

# Usefulness

As may be inferred from its physiological action, Coca as a remedial agent is adapted to a wide sphere of usefulness, and if we accept the hypothesis that the influence of Coca is to free the blood from waste and to repair tissue, we have a ready explanation of its action. Bartholow says:"
"It is probable that some of the constituents of Coca are utilized in the economy as food, and that the retardation of tissue-waste is not the sole reason why work may be done by its use which can not be done by the same person

*Coca as a remedial agent* without it." Stockmann
*is adapted to a wide* considers that the source
*sphere of usefulness.* of endurance from Coca
can hardly depend solely
upon the stimulation of the
nervous system, but that there must at the same time be an
economizing in the bodily exchange.

An idea which is further confirmed by the total absence
of emaciation or other injurious consequences in the Indians who constantly use Coca. He suggests that Coca may
possibly diminish the consumption of carbohydrates by
the muscles during exertion. If this is so, then less oxygen would be required, and there is an explanation of the
influence of Coca in relieving breathlessness in ascending
mountains.

Prominent in the application of Coca is its antagonism
to the alcohol and opium habit. Freud, of Vienna, considers that Coca not only allays the craving for morphine, but
that relapses do not occur. Coca certainly will check the
muscle racking pains incidental to abandonment of opium
by an habitue, and its use is well indicated in the condition
following the abuse of alcohol when the stomach can not
digest food. It not only allays the necessity for food, but
removes the distressing nervous phenomena. Dr. Bauduy,
of St. Louis, early called the attention of the American
Neurological Association to the efficiency of Coca in the
treatment of melancholia, and the benefit of Coca in a long
list of nervous or nerveless conditions has been extolled
by a host of physicians. Shoemaker, of Philadelphia, has
advocated the external use of Coca in eczema, dermatitis,
herpes, rosacea, urticaria and allied conditions where an
application of the Fluid Extract of Coca one part to four of
water lends a sedative action to the skin.

The influence of Coca on the pulse and temperature
has suggested its employment in collapse and weak heart
as recommended by Da Costa, and it has been favorably

employed to relieve dropsy depending on debility of the
heart, and for uraemia and scanty secretion of urine. In
seasickness Coca acts as a prophylactic as well as a remedy.
Vomiting of pregnancy may be arrested by cocaine administered either by the mouth or rectum. In the debility of fevers Coca has been found especially serviceable, and in this
connection Dr. A. R. Booth, of the Marine Hospital Service,
at Shreveport, Louisiana, has written me that he considers
cocaine one of the most valuable aids in the treatment of
yellow fever. [1] By controlling nausea and vomiting, [2] as
a cardiac stimulant, [3] as a haemostatic when indicated,
[4] to hold in abeyance hunger, which at times would be
intolerable but for the effect of cocaine. One who has seen
a yellow fever stomach, especially from a subject who has
died from "black vomit," must have been impressed with
the absolute impossibility of such an organ performing its
physiological functions.

Dr. Booth makes it an inflexible rule, never to allow
a yellow fever patient food by the mouth until convales-
cence is well established. In cases of fine physique he has
kept the patient without food for ten or twelve days, and
in two cases fourteen and fifteen days respectively, solely
by the judicious administration of cocaine in tablets by
the mouth. Of two hundred and six cases of yellow fever
treated in this manner there was not one relapse. A similar
use is made of cocaine to abate the canine hunger of certain
cases of epilepsy and insanity, as well as to appease thirst
in diabetes.

The.Peruvian Indians employ Coca to stimulate uter-
ine contractions and regard it as a powerful aphrodisiac.
Leopold Casper, of Berlin, considers Coca one of the best
of genital tonics, and many modern observers concur in
this opinion.[40] Vecki[47] says that cocaine internally to a man
aged fifty-six invariably occasioned sexual excitement and
cheerfulness. The Homoeopaths who have long regarded
Coca as a valuable remedy, employ Coca in sexual excess-

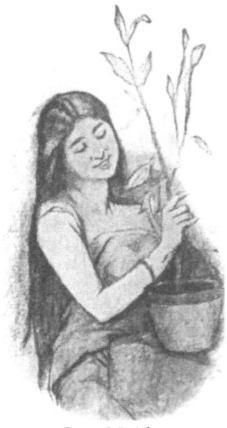

*Coca Maiden*

es, especially when dependent on onanism. Allen has given a "proving" of Coca that covers twelve pages, and Hering's Materia Medica gives provings by twenty-four persons, and recommends Coca in troubles coming with a low state of the barometer. Hempel says: "I have found a remarkable aversion to exertion of any kind in consequence of nervous exhaustion frequently relieved with great promptness by Coca." But it is not my intention to here enumerate the various symptoms for which Coca is regarded as a specific.

I have only space to briefly suggest it possible application as a remedy. A resume of the various conditions in which Coca has commonly been found serviceable, and its relative employment as classified from the experience of several hundred physicians, correspondents in this research, will be found tabulated in the appendix. Coca may be given in doses equivalent to one or two drachms of the leaves three or four times a day, either as an infusion or as a fluid extract or wine; the latter especially being serviceable for support in acute disease as well as an adjunct indicated in those conditions where its use may tend to maintain the balance of health.

# Excessive Doses

It is a noteworthy fact already referred to, that there has been no recorded case of poisoning from Coca, nor cases of Coca addiction commonly regarded as "habit." The cases of cocaine poisoning and addiction often sensationally reported are even open to grave doubt. The condition termed "cocaine habit" is not generally accepted by physicians, as shown in the specific report in the appendix. Certainly the very general use of cocaine as an anassthetic has not resulted relatively in anything like the number of rare accidents from the use of chloroform and ether, and this fact must appear the more remarkable when it is appreciated that chloroform and ether are administered under skilled observation, while cocaine is commonly employed by hundreds of thousands—even millions—of laymen, many of whom are absolutely ignorant of its properties.

*There has been no recorded case of poisoning from Coca, nor cases of Coca addiction commonly regarded as "habit."*

The use of any alkaloid should be with the appreciation that the factor of personal idiosyncrasy may exert an influence to occasion irregular action. A case of fatal poisoning has been recorded against cocaine from as small a dose as two-thirds of a grain of the hydrochlorate given hypo-dermic-ally, and from twenty minims of a four per cent, solution (four-fifths of a grain) of the same salt injected into the urethra, and smaller doses it is asserted have produced alarming symptoms. On the other hand, numerous cases are recorded where excessive doses of the alkaloid have been continued for long periods without giving rise to serious trouble. A recovery is recorded after forty-six grains of cocaine had been taken into the stomach, and in one case twenty-three grains of cocaine was used hypodermically daily.

Dr. William A. Hammond experimented upon himself by injecting cocaine subcutaneously. Commencing with one grain the dose was gradually increased until eighteen grains were taken in four portions within five minutes of each other. His pulse increased to one hundred and forty and became irregular. Five minutes after the last injection he felt elated and utterly regardless of surroundings, consciousness being lost within half an hour. The next morning on going to his study where the experiment had been performed he found the floor strewn with books of reference and the chairs overturned, indicating there had been an active mental and physical excitement. He had turned off the gas, gone upstairs to bed, lighted the gas in his sleeping apartment and retired quite as had been his custom.

At nine o'clock the following morning he woke with a splitting headache, and experienced considerable cardiac and respiratory disturbance, and for several days after felt the effects of his indiscretion by languor and indisposition to mental or physical exertion and difficulty in concentration of attention. He considered that eighteen grains of cocaine was nearly a fatal dose for him, and if he had taken it in one dose instead of within twenty minutes it might have been disastrous. This experimenter did not observe any influence upon the ganglia at the base of the brain. There was no disturbance of sensibility, no anaesthesia nor hyperesthesia, nor interference with motility except some muscles of the face, which were subject to slight twitching.

There were no hallucinations. Dr. Hammond asserted that there is no such thing as a "cocaine habit." He had given cocaine to many patients, both male and female, and never had a single objection to the alkaloid being discontinued, not as much trouble in ceasing its use, in fact, as there would have been to give up tea or coffee, and nothing like so much as to have abandoned alcohol or tobacco. He personally used for a nasal affection, during four

months, from sixteen to twenty grains a day, averaging
about six hundred grains of cocaine a month, applied in
solution to the mucous membrane of the nose. During this
period he experienced slight mental exhilaration and some
indisposition to sleep. Subsequently he used nearly eight
hundred grains within thirty-five days. In each instance the
drug was discontinued without the slightest difficulty.

# Influence of Cocaine

Dr. Caudwell, of London, experimented upon himself with
both Coca and cocaine. He took increasing doses of fluid extract of Coca until two ounces were taken at a dose.
From this he experienced giddiness with unsteadiness of
gait, followed by sensations of mental and physical activity
when it seemed any exertion could have been undertaken
without difficulty. Under cocaine, in doses of one grain he
experienced drowsiness, followed by sleep, and then persistent insomnia. Two and a half grains produced frontal
headache, mental excitement and marked insomnia. Three
grains after abstinence from food for twenty-four hours
produced drowsiness, slight vertigo and wakefulness with
a sense of well being. On the following morning five grains
produced giddiness with a supra-orbital headache and a
sense of weight at the pit of the stomach, while the pupils
were widely dilated, and there was inability for exertion.

All unpleasant sensations following this experiment
had passed in two hours, though dilatation of the pupils
lasted for six hours. Professor Bignon, of Lima, considers
that the Peruvian Indians consume daily an amount of
Coca which represents from thirty to forty centigrammes—
[4.5 to 6. grains] of cocaine. He regards ten centigrammes
of that alkaloid per day [1.5 grains] a good average dose
for those unaccustomed to its use. The average initial dose
of cocaine hypodermically should not exceed a quarter of a
grain. Under a moderate dose of cocaine, the central ner-

*Under a poisonous dose of cocaine there is an initial increase of respiration and of the heart beat, both of which soon slow under the influence of paralysis of the vaso motor center.*

vous system is stimulated through a direct action on the nerve cells. There is psychic exaltation, with increased capacity for mental work, which passes off in a few hours and is followed by complete restoration to the normal condition without after depression. Indeed, whatever depression there may be precedes the exaltation. From larger doses, the medulla and the sensory columns of the spinal cord may be directly affected, but only after very large doses is there weakness and lassitude, and general anaesthesia can only follow from an excessive dose.

Under a poisonous dose of cocaine there is an initial increase of respiration and of the heart beat, both of which soon slow under the influence of paralysis of the vaso motor center, this effect of cocaine upon respiration and the circulation being similar to that from atropine. The pupils are widely dilated and do not respond to light. Involuntary movement of the muscles of mastication, as in chewing, and rotation of the head or body has been noted in animals. There may be epileptiform attacks, clonic convulsions or tetanus.

# Symptoms of Poisoning

The most common symptoms of cocaine poisoning are those of profound prostration, with dyspnoea, pallor, cyanosis and sweat. When the drug has been taken by the stomach that organ should be evacuated and washed out, while in any case stimulants may be indicated, such as nitrite of amyl, ammonia, ether hypo-dermically, chloroform to check spasm of the respiratory muscles and even

artificial respiration may be indicated. After the severe
symptoms have passed chloral may be administered.
Both chloral and morphine are regarded as antagonistic to
cocaine. Recovery may take place even after a long period
of unconsciousness. I was called in one case to a dentist's
office to resuscitate a patient after his careless injection of
an unknown quantity of cocaine, and we labored over the
subject eight hours before consciousness was restored.

Mosso puts the lethal dose of cocaine at 0.03 per kilo-
gramme, in animals, and in man it is probably less. Mann-
heim, from a collection of about a hundred cases of cocaine
poisoning—of which nine were fatal—has determined that
one gramme [15.43 grains], of the alkaloid may be considered a fatal dose in man. A "cocaine habit," as already referred to, is not generally accepted. Yet symptoms presumably due to the excessive use of large doses of cocaine are
described. These embrace frequency of pulse, relaxation of
the arterial system, profuse perspiration, rapid fall of flesh
and hallucinations of sight or feeling. A peculiar symptom
of chronic cocaine poisoning is that known as Magnan's
symptom, after the name of the describer. It is an hallucina-
tion of sensation in which the patient complains of feeling
a foreign body under the skin. While other hallucinations
are common from poisons this is said to be distinctive of
cocaine.

There is but one further feature in the physiological
study of Coca that we have to consider, and that is the
manner of its elimination from the body. From experiments
of Dr. Helm-sing it was long since determined that cocaine
is very difficult of detection in animal tissues. This may be
appreciated when the important role, which it is possible
that Coca plays in assimilation is considered. When taken
into the stomach Coca soon disappears from the alimentary canal, being decomposed and gradually setting free the
products to which its physiological action is due. As these
several alkaloids are carried through the tissues, they enter

into further chemical change whereby they are still further broken down, and only soon after the administration of a very large dose is it possible to recover the bases from the alkaline urine with benzoyl. Immediately after a poisonous dose of cocaine given to a cat there was found a distinctive reaction in the urine and blood, but a diminished dose gave after a longer interval only faint tracings, which gradually disappeared.

Because of this difficulty of detection the decomposition products of Coca, chiefly as ecgonine, are determined post-mortem by a process of assay. The comminuted tissue is mixed with two parts of acidulated alcohol and digested at 60° in a reflux condenser, the process being repeated with fresh alcohol and the filtrates evaporated to almost dryness. The residue is taken up with water, and the solution shaken out with ether, the residual concentrated liquid being precipitated with baryta and extracted repeatedly with ether. The ethereal solution is then evaporated in a vacuum and the residue tested for the alkaloid.

The fact that the Coca products are so thoroughly consumed in the body indicates the important influence these substances exercise in nutrition, the philosophy of which has been more fully detailed in other chapters.

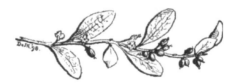

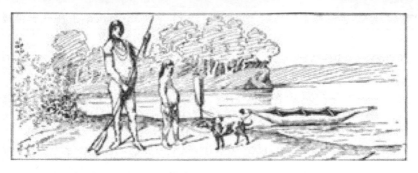

## Chapter 9

# Coca As a Food

URING the ages that Coca has been employed, its use as a source of energy and endurance without other means of subsistence, long since gave rise to the problem whether Coca can rightly be considered a food. Associated with this thought, there has apparently been suggested to the minds of some a name of similar sound of more common usage. The mention of Coca in a food connection has at once recalled to them cocoa and chocolate, which, though often components of an excellent dietary, are in no manner whatever related to Coca even by the most distant ties of kinship. This similarity of names has occasioned amusing errors, some of which are related— without reflection on their authors—to impress the distinction. Cocoa is prepared from the roasted seeds of the palm *Theohroma Cacao*, Linn., an ancient tree of tropical America, the product of which was early introduced by the Spaniards to the Old World. It belongs to the order Sterculiacece, of which the African kola—(Sterculia), is a relative. The name cocoa has been adapted from the less euphonious specific term cacao of the genus Theobroma, while chocolate—which is prepared from cacao—is a word of Mexican derivation, from choco—cacao, and latl—water, referring to its preparation as a beverage. From cocoa there is obtained an active principle present in the proportion of about two per cent. This, first described by Woskresensky in 1845, was named theobromine, and though not identical, has been found closely allied to caffeine. From phonetic semblance Coca has been erroneously associated with cocoa or with the coconut, just as these latter two have been misquoted by the unthinking. Thus Dr. Johnson in his Dictionary published in 1755, confoundedthem, as emphasized in the following quotation which he has given under cocoa:

> "Amid those orchards of the Sun, Give me to drain the *cocoa's* milky bowl, And from the palm to draw its freshening wine!"
> —Thomson, *Seasons*, (Summer)

Those who have followed the history of Coca, and the story of the gradual unfolding of its leaves to usefulness, may express a cunning surprise that so careless a confusion of terms is possible. Some may consider that such knowledge is purely technical and hardly to be expected of the laity, yet very many of the medical profession are apparently among those who are uninformed. To an exceedingly large class Coca means simply chocolate, while the coconut is erroneously regarded as belonging to the same botanical group. Certain knowing ones there are who appreciate that cocoa seeds yield chocolate; yet among these some few are content in a belief that the leaf of the cocoa plant is the Coca chewed bj the Andean Indians. It is hardly to be expected that physicians, who are commonly regarded as well informed, would continue an ignorance on this subject, in view of the very wide interest awakened by the application of cocaine.

In spite of the antiquity of centuries, the fact remains that Coca is not well known. This has been emphasized in the present inquiry. That this is not a mere apparent error, through hasty or illegible orthography, may be assured from the fullness of certain replies. Some of these, after describing the physiological action and therapeutic uses of Coca, have displayed a confusional state of knowledge by saying they have used some preparation of breakfast cocoa in place of tea or coffee at meals, or in greater detail have said: "I never use the liquid preparations—I prefer chocolate." One enthusiast, from a personal examination of cocoa with a microscope, pronounced "it free from adulteration," and another busy practitioner who uses "the ordinary cocoa of commerce for drinking at the table," and to whom some vague recollections of former readings has entwined the change of Coca by age with an awe inspiring potency of its active principle, says: "It should be seen to that it is fresh; age causes it to deteriorate," and concludes: "It is a dangerous remedy, which should be used with caution."

One has answered my physiological question: "From memory, of the personal effects from the use of sweet chocolate." Another really kindly disposed gentleman regrets: "The great diversity of opinion regarding the effects in the application of the medicine," and as an explanation of his own neglect cites as illustration: "I am very unpleasantly affected by coffee or tea, presumably by caffeine. It depresses my heart's action and delays digestion. Ordinarily breakfast coffee for two mornings makes my pulse intermit ; strong tea the same. Cocoa or chocolate is something worse. It does not digest, causing unpleasant eructations and a heavy, sour feeling in my stomach. Most people like cocoa, or especially chocolate, and prefer it when ill to coffee. From personal dislike I never recommend it and have never investigated the good qualities ascribed to it."

Amidst such a jumble resulting from an investigation among those especially educated to be observers it seems easier to believe with what seriousness the article was written some few years ago on *Cocoa and Cocaine,* a title which might be overlooked as a typographical error were it not

*There was early desire on the part of the Church to discountenance the use of Coca, whether it contained food properties or not, because of its superstitious associations.*

for the statement that "cocoa contains two alkaloids, theobromine and cocaine,"[1] while a further muddle is possible through the recent introduction of a cocoa preparation by an English firm called "Cocoaine." There is always confusion unavoidable in the gradual evolvement of any remedy to usefulness; in the present instance this has not been confined to any one department, but has extended through each branch of research from the doings of the early Spanish historians to the botanists, the chemists, physiologists and physicians.

All the accounts of the early writers of Andean travel indicate that Coca has a phenomenal effect upon endurance, so great, indeed, that many of these accounts have been regarded as simply fabulous; but as we have considered the possibilities of Coca through the potential energy hidden in its leaf, it is very easy to trace the foundation of truth from these stories. The Indians were described as relying upon Coca for food and drink, with no other resource. "If you ask them why they thus continually keep Coca in the mouth and venerate it, they will answer you that its use prevents the feeling of hunger, thirst, and loss of strength, as well as preserves them in health." Cieza refers to Coca as a most marvellous panacea "against hunger, or any need of food or drink."

There was early desire on the part of the Church to discountenance the use of Coca, whether it contained food properties or not, because of its superstitious associations. Its use must be prohibited because it was a substance "which is connected with the work of idolatry and sorcery, strengthening the wicked in their delusions, and asserted by every competent judge to possess no true virtues; but on the contrary, to cause the deaths of innumerable Indians, while it ruins the health of the few who survive." So that in order to restore the usefulness of Coca to the Indian, to whom it was found a necessity by his Spanish masters, this law was repealed after it had been demonstrated for politic reasons that Coca could not be a food. Some of the earlier writers presumed that any sustaining action must be due to some starchy or mucilaginous properties in the leaf, and to maintain this hypothesis it was asserted that every ounce of leaves yielded a half ounce of gum. Poeppig, who has written many hasty conclusions of Coca, denied this, because from repeated analysis he found such a small portion of mucilage in the leaf that its food properties must be slight. He said: "The saliva of the Coca chewer is thin and watery, like that which flows from the chewing of tobacco, and it betrays not the least trace of sugar to the palate."

# Prejudice of Doubt

Through all obstacles of prejudice or doubt the facts of the sustaining influence of Coca are so apparent as to be undeniable, and skepticism must be carried very far to now doubt the effect of Coca on nutrition. As Dr. Weddell has said: "One of two things is certain. Either the Coca contains some nutritive principle which directly sustains the strength or it does not contain it, and therefore simply deceives hunger while acting on the system." He was of the opinion that the nutritive principle of Coca might be due to the presence of a notable quantity of nitrogen, together with assimilable carbonized products.

This same hesitancy between acknowledging effects which are apparent to all observers, united with a preformed prejudice without the weight of scientific evidence, is still intermixed in the confusion of our own time. An indication of the readiness with which opinion is swayed may be inferred from some of the letters received in my investigation. One physician writes: "I quit the use of Coca after some publications in the journals. I was scared off too soon, probably." This conservatism, born of timidity, is shown through many replies similar to the following: "I scarcely ever prescribe a medicine unless it has been done by others more venturesome than myself; I think the hesitancy in prescribing Coca was owing to the numerous reports of the cocaine habit contracted by patients which have been published from time to time;" yet such so-called "habit," as elsewhere shown, is not proven.

"We have seen under what difficulty the Andeans were permitted to continue the use of Coca as a means of sustenance, and from that early superstition to the subsequent prejudice and confusion, which has continued even to our own time, it is not at all surprising that Coca has been little understood, wrongly applied, or has occasioned little thought toward its application as a food.

The popular idea of the term food may possibly be embodied in the one word—repletion—without regard to whether the substance consumed is capable in itself to sustain the bodily functions. It is such a thought perhaps which prompted the reply to my inquiry as to the dietetic uses of Coca: "This is all a terrible mistake—cocoa is used as food, but Coca, never!" The misconception of the term food, as well as the mistaken application arising from this, has laid the foundation for many a disease. Scientists well know that there is no one article of food that will supply all the requirements of the organism. Nature demands a certain quantity of chemical elements, properly apportioned and combined, which shall go to repair the tissues. It is by this repeated aid that the complex process of living in the struggle for the maintenance of supremacy or of even mere existence, is continued.

*The popular idea of the term food may possibly be embodied in the one word—repletion.*

The whole matter of dietetics is little understood—not among those whose duty it is to explain such matters, but among the people who eat indiscriminately of whatever may be offered so long as it shall be of tempting form and palatable, and to whom the ponderable is commonly the more potent. This is often the occasion for much resultant misery, poor health, and consequent unhappiness, generated through an improper use of those blessings which are given to enjoy. It is use without abuse that should be impressed—not abstinence, and yet not unbridled indulgence. Some who look at this narrowly are apt to moralize, as did the little chap when deprived of his sweets and forced to castor oil: "All the good things *is* bad, and all the bad things *is* good." The fact is we become so familiarized with ordinary functions that their performance is often lightly dismissed as instinctive—something which every one should know for himself. As a result few care to read physiology while well, and when they are ill it is too late.

In a modern civilization desire is apt to seek indulgence in proportion to opportunity. There is a privilege in wealth, increase of which usually suggests freer methods, and greater comforts, which often point toward sensual indulgence rather than to any philosophy of living. Then follows not only luxuriance, but an extravagance and ultimate *dis-ease,* a veritable want of ease and comfort. This has ever been the cycle since the world began, and it rolls on so easily and quickly that before excesses are even dreamed of much constitutional harm is done. But: "the doctors are here to attend to such little matters; let them do the worrying, we will continue our enjoyment."

The history of all aboriginal peoples indicates a simple dietary of natural products, a thought from which our vegetarian friends doubtless find much prestige:—"*The field as yet untitled, their feasts afford And fill a sumptuous and unenvied board.*" sang Hesiod. We have seen how the Incans lived largely upon maize or the starchy food of various

tubers; yet while the common herd must find content in
these, the nobility enriched their feasts with game and
the various productions from the hot valleys and stimulated their desires or allayed the effects of over indulgence
by Coca. Even fresh fish was served at the royal tables,
brought by rapid runners, who by a special grant of a few
handfuls of Coca were enabled to make a trip of several
hundred miles from the sea to the imperial city of Cuzco in
a single day.

# Growth of Dietetics

It is curious to consider how the first blind selections of
foodstuffs may have been made in the early days when
there were no botanists, chemists nor cooks. Many must
have chosen wrongly and suffered for their boldness, for
we know that similar errors are occurring about us everywhere and with equally unfortunate results. These early
errors gave rise to the necessity for a more careful choice—
for an elective knowledge, and we who followed long ages
after, while continuing to profit by the methods of these
early specialists benefit through their method of natural selection. We owe gratitude for a multitude of important and
what are now considered absolutely necessary foodstuffs
which have been preserved and improved for us through
a refinement of cultivation and are now universally used.
Among these we have examples in those Peruvian products, Coca, maize and the potato, which have been so long
cultivated that the most profound research has not been
enabled to determine their original home in the wild state.

We have seen why it is probable that aboriginal peoples were vegetarians, and we know through the ancient
historians that the use of meat was often considered un-
lawful or unholy. Possibly the use of meat may be associated with the stimulus demanded in the incessant struggle
for supremacy in the larger cities where statistics show

its greater consumption than among agricultural people. Homer alludes to the moderate use of meat among his heroes, a chine of beef roasted being a favorite dish not often indulged in. Boiled meats and broths seem to have been among the earlier means of using flesh, but as tastes change, so these early simple methods soon gave place to greater variety. Then—as the senses have ever led the judgment—we read of wealthy gourmands who vied with each other in serving absurd and often disgusting dishes as epicurean delights. Apicius—who wished for the neck of a stork that he might longer enjoy the delights of deglutition —dissolved pearls and offered them in wine to his guests, and after squandering a fortune in dining killed himself because he had but a paltry eighty thousand pounds left.

Among some of the dainty relishes served during the early Grecian period was the dormouse, the hedgehog and puppies, while the flesh of the young ass was considered a delicacy. Peacocks were regarded as essential to every well ordered banquet, and Aufidius Lures is said to have derived an income of many thousands of dollars from the sale of these at a price of seven to eleven dollars apiece. Such fabulous sums were spent for single entertainments that Seneca, who was himself enormously wealthy, refers to the profusion of dishes and extravagance of the times when he alludes to:

> "Vitellius' table which did hold
> As many creatures as the ark of old."

The Middle Ages were scarcely better in habits of indulgence ; swans, peacocks and the wild boar continued among the delicacies of the table until long after the reign of Edward the Fourth, while Charles the Fifth of Germany was a royal gourmand who delighted in dishes quite as extravagant as any of those that graced the tables of the Greeks or Romans, some of his viands being lizard soup, roast horse and cats in jelly, which were washed down with deep draughts of Rhine wine.

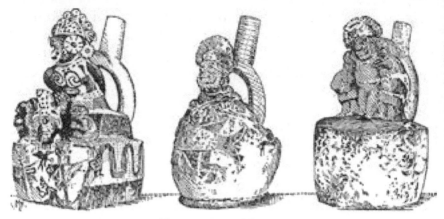

### *Peruvian Vases*

We have seen that among the Incas hospitality was considered so essential as to demand a law necessitating and governing its practice. On all state occasions the monarch feasted the nobles at a banquet, where important consummations were solemnized by royal bumpers of the native *chicha* quaffed from golden goblets. Among the masses the usual hours for eating were eight or nine in the morning and at sunset; these latter periods Garcilasso says were sometimes turned into a' veritable revelry extending far into the night, a custom which has not been wholly neglected among the modern Andeans, who were quick to adopt the *fiesta* which is prompted on slight impulse in all Spanish countries.

# Appetite vs. Opportunity

If we review the history of dietetics we shall find it fluctuating between indulgence and satiety, with an occasional interim of enforced fasting through necessity. During the last century many were actually starved through the return wave of abstemiousness, because of the scientific efforts of their medical advisers, many of whom—like Dr. Sangrado,[7] urged copious draughts of hot water with liberal blood letting, or insisted on some rigid dietary for all, unmindful of the fact that what might be advisable for a sick man may not prove desirable to one in health. Thus matters dietetical have largely balanced themselves through appetite and opportunity, while physicians have too commonly followed the methods of the masses and suffered or benefited in accordance with the resources of their environment.

With such changes between excess and abstemiousness— of too much or too little advice—popular views have naturally been unsettled or indifferent on the diet question. It is unanimous upon one point, however, and as Sancho Panza,[8] after he became Governor of the Island of Barataria—"Having appetite, must eat something." It is to teach what this something may be which proves the great stumbling block. It can only be broadly done in any book, the individual necessities must be the subject of personal attention.

One value of knowledge is to recognize error; it is negative as well as affirmative. In matters dietetic there should be sufficient preliminary education to understand more closely not only what to eat with advantage but what to avoid in order to make better citizens. We are at present in an age of preventive methods of many things, and it would seem that the modern physician—he who aims more especially to guide his patients so as to keep them from becoming ill, rather than he who confines his problems to curing them when prostrate— may find the greatest and most profitable solution in the maintenance of health through an appropriate and well directed dietary. Without necessarily following we can adapt the means of others which seem desirable to our own necessities. If in this adaption prejudice be set aside and the possibilities of Coca shall be considered, there will occur opportunities which must ultimately result in a more pronounced benefit to overworked and overtired humanity.

It is only within the last fifty years that our chemi-
co-physiologic knowledge in dietetics has developed from
the foundation laid by Liebig, the work since his time
tending chiefly to clearing up errors or explaining his theories, which are not yet fully accepted. From a review of the
opinion of many physiologists it is difficult to give a concise definition of a food. In accordance with the theory here
advocated I will thus define it: *Food is any substance taken
into the body which maintains integrity of the tissues and creates
the energy we term life.* With such a definition in view, it may
the more readily be appreciated that it is not necessarily
what is eaten but what is assimilated that is beneficial. It is
somewhat as Froude has said of knowledge: "The knowledge which a man can use is the only real knowledge." So
the food which the body utilizes is the only real food. This
of necessity must vary with conditions and environment,
and as civilization tends to shape all things to her own
demands, it is the object of dietetics to adapt the varying
possibilities to man's requirements.

# Object of Food

It is a common assertion advanced in all seriousness that
one partakes of the nature of the food eaten. The vegetarian claims to see in the meat eater the ferocity of the
carnivorous animal. The pugnacious beef-eating Briton
and the seemingly docile Chinese rice-eater are sometimes
cited as examples. Aside from the effect on the emotions
as a result of companionship there can be no weight to the
homely saying: "He who drinks beer thinks beer." Again,
the idea that: "Every part strengthens a part" is another
common error, for physiologically we know that bone does
not make bone nor does fat make fat. There are many who
presume that vegetables are the only appropriate food
for man. Plutarch tells us that Grillus—who, according
to the doctrine of transmigration, had at one time been a

beast—describes how much better he fed and lived when an animal than when he was turned again to man. It is not necessary to accept this literally, but it suggests the fact that all flesh is grass and emphasizes the indestructibility of matter. But man need not eat grass as did Nebuchadnezzar, for when he eats animal flesh he virtually eats the very elements which are comprised in the vegetable kingdom and which have been appropriately elaborated.

Our tissues are a combination of chemical elements, chief among which are carbon, hydrogen, oxygen and nitrogen, with some minor ones present as salts in small proportions. These elements compose all animal cells, just as we have seen their presence is essential in vegetable structures.

In order that the integrity of the tissues shall be maintained these principles must be intro-

*Chemistry teaches us that energy is liberated by every chemical union, and so it is the conversion of the food materials taken and containing these chemical elements which liberates the energy essential to continue the cell growth which constitutes existence.*

duced into the organism. It has been estimated that the average daily loss of these consists of carbon, 281.2 grammes; hydrogen, 6.3 grammes; oxygen, 681.41 grammes; nitrogen, 18.8 grammes, so that the selection of any dietary should be made to approximate this proportionate loss in order to balance waste. These elements are not of themselves food, nor can they synthetically be built into a food in the laboratory.

Chemistry teaches us that energy is liberated by every chemical union, and so it is the conversion of the food materials taken and containing these chemical elements which liberates the energy essential to continue the cell growth which constitutes existence. The body is but a colony of cells through which the several elements pass after an elaboration from inorganic compounds through vegetable and animal tissue. After their property is exerted to the maintenance of a higher organization they are cast aside, only to again pass through the cycle of elaboration and to be again consumed and so on for innumerable times without ultimate loss, but in each interchange yielding the energy we term life.

Pood substances according to variation of primal elements are embraced in two groups: The nitrogenous—of which albumen is the type—containing carbon, hydrogen, oxygen and nitrogen, comprises the proteids of which muscle and the structure of the body generally is formed, which among foods is represented by the lean of meat, fish and poultry, casein of milk and cheese, albumen of eggs, gelatin, gluten of cereals and the albuminous substance contained in such vegetables as peas, beans and lentils. The second class, the non-nitrogenous—technically known as the carbohydrates—contains carbon, hydrogen and oxygen and embraces the sugars and starches, however derived, and the oils and fats whether of cream, flesh, fish or fowl.

The nitrogenous group constitutes the incombustible framework of the body, in which, according to Liebig, the second class—the combustible non-nitrogenous—fuel foods are consumed. It seems strange to speak of combustion, which is suggestive of fire, as going on within the body, but the process of chemical conversion within is akin to that of combustion without, and before food can reach its ultimate end in the repair of tissue, internal oxidation is essential to create heat, which is an index of the available force for work. The deprivation of food is chiefly made manifest through heat loss, and starvation has been paralleled to death by cold, while in restoration from prolonged lack of food the application of warmth is at first really more essential than is food.

From various physiological experiments it has been shown that animals fed exclusively on a non-nitrogenous diet speedily emaciate and die, as though from starvation, and experimentally life is more prolonged in those fed with nitrogenous than in those fed upon non-nitrogenous food, while animal heat is maintained fully as well by the former as by the latter.[10] Most of the evils of mankind are due to mal-nutri-tion, whereby the body undergoes changes which are comparable to those resulting either from starvation or from overproduction. Changes which are really induced not necessarily by taking too much or too little food, but from taking improper proportions of the two broad classes, or due to a lack of stimulus to a proper conversion. At times the excess will pass through the alimentary canal unchanged or remain in the intestine unabsorbed, undergoing a slow decomposition setting free gases and inducing various digestive disturbances.

# Food Conversion

The carbohydrates are readily converted into storage food, which, under certain conditions, may be transformed into fat, and this may so clog the working of the organs as to prove a decided detriment to the body rather than a source of strength. It is commonly considered, however, that an excess of nitrogenous food is the chief source of trouble in overfeeding, and possibly, because of concentration, this class of food may the more readily be eaten in excess unthinkingly.

There is a vast physiological importance to the alimentary canal, for through it is introduced all the material which goes to build up the organism, including every chemical element of the body except oxygen. Hippocrates considered that the stomach bears the same relation to animals as soil does to plants, a parallel which leads a modern writer[11] to say: "A man whose digestion is defective is comparable to a tree which planted in sterile soil finishes by withering and perishing." The alimentary canal, however, does not end at the stomach, an organ which is really a mere expanded reservoir for the digestive tract. The fact that conversion and absorption takes place through almost the entire extent of this canal is not commonly considered. There seems to prevail a popular idea that it is the stomach only which is responsible in preparing food for assimilation. This opinion was so prevalent in the time of Dr. William Hunter that he remarked the error by saying to his class: "Gentlemen, physiologists will have it that the stomach is a mill; others that it is a fermenting vat; others again that it is a stew-pan; but in my view of the matter it is neither a mill, a fermenting vat nor a stew-pan, but a stomach, gentleman, a stomach."

To effect the proper conversion of food its minute division is essential in order that the several digestive substances with which the bolus comes in contact in its passage through the alimentary canal may act upon the different parts for which they have an elective affinity. By the action of these enzymes, or ferments as they are termed, the food is rendered soluble, and so made capable of absorption. A substance taken as food which remains insoluble is virtually out of the body so far as nutrition is concerned and is really only an irritant. The whole process of digestion is one of solution so that the food may pass through the tissues into the blood. Absorption takes place in every part of the digestive tract and as the unabsorbed mass is passed onward different ferments act upon different portions of the bolus to prepare it for solution. The process of mastication when properly performed not only breaks up the food and softens the mass with saliva ready for its transit, but sets free a ferment which changes the insoluble starchy particles into a soluble sugar. The flow of saliva is increased by the act of chewing, or may even be effected reflexly by the emotions through the sympathetic nerve, either of which causes in creases the blood supply to the secreting gland.

There is an increased flow of saliva from chewing Coca which is not wholly dependent upon mastication, but the function is increased through physiological action. This may be the starting point of its beneficial influence in the conversion of starchy foods which is ultimately pronouncedly effective in the building up of muscular tissue. Then through its action upon the gastric secretions Coca furthers the digestive process instead of checking it by any an aesthetic action on the stomach, as has been erroneously suggested and as is commonly supposed.

In this relation Dr. Weddle says: "I can affirm very positively that Coca, as it is taken habitually, does not satiate hunger. This is a fact of which I have convinced myself by daily experience. The Indians who accompanied me on my journey chewed Coca during the whole day, but at evening they filled their stomachs like fasting men, and I am certain I have seen one devour as much food at a single meal as I should have consumed during two days."

# The Hunger Sense

A host of modern observers have recognized the true food Value of Coca in nutrition, particularly serviceable in the emergency of protracted fevers or in debility until other food may take its place, and life has been prolonged for long periods under the exclusive use of Coca during the enforced abstinence from other food.* Rusby found that Coca allays the hunger sense, but does not suspend ability, being really a tonic to digestion, while Reichert, from laboratory experiments, concluded that Coca might not only replace food, but "in cases of restricted diet, or even in the entire absence of food, will enable the individual to perform as much or even more work than under ordinary circumstances."[12]

There has been an attempt to explain this influence of Coca upon the sense of hunger through an anassthetic action on the mucous membrane of the stomach, which seems parallel to the idea that tobacco abolishes the sense of hunger through disgust by prostrating nervous action. But as Anstie says: "It is wholly improbable that agents having a depressing influence on the nervous system, such as antimony and ipecac, would relieve the feeling of weakness occasioned through hunger and fatigue."[13] It should be recalled that the sense of hunger is not local, but general. It is the demand of the system for nourishment, a call for fuel in order to supply energy.

The sensation is experienced by the stomach reflexly, but the demand may be fulfilled by the introduction of food into the organism through any channel. Thus the sensation of thirst which is commonly referred to a dryness in the throat may be relieved by the addition of fluid to the blood by any method. The probability is that Coca through its nitrogenous influence so affects metabolism as to enable the organism to utilize substances which might otherwise pass off as waste. Just as we have seen in plant structures a similar influence under well-apportioned nitrogenous substances.

The local effect on the stomach by the introduction of food is to cause the mucous membrane to become reddened through an increased blood supply. This stimulates the gastric secretion of watery fluid, salts, pepsin and the acids which render that ferment active. The action on starch which commenced in the mouth is now checked and the solution of saline particles of the food is continued, while the insoluble nitrogenous bodies are converted into soluble peptones. The gastric juice also acts by retarding decomposition

*The local effect on the stomach by the introduction of food is to cause the mucous membrane to become reddened through an increased blood supply.*

in bodies which are prone to this change in the presence of warmth and moisture.

From the stomach the food mass passes to the small intestine, where the influence of the gastric fluid ceases and a new process is commenced by the bile, intestinal juice, and the secretions of the pancreas, acting in an alkaline fluid. Here the albuminous materials which have escaped the former processes are converted into soluble peptones, while any starchy matters which have not been converted by the ptyaline of the saliva are also acted upon and changed into glucose. The pancreatic juice also emulsifies the oils and fats, splitting them up into their fatty acids and glycerine to enable their more ready absorption by the lacteals of the intestine and by the blood vessels.

Food does not pass through the digestive tract just as a weight might be dropped through a tube, but having once entered the (esophagus it is propelled by a peculiar undulating movement termed peristalsis—a motion similar to the method by which an angle worm creeps along. The muscular fibres contract and draw a portion of the tube over the mass to be propelled, elongation then takes place and a succession of such waves rather draws the substance down than presses it on, while at the same time it is checked from too rapid passage, so that digestion may proceed.

As the mass reaches the large intestine there is probably no digestive process continued, though assimilation may take place through the absorption of some portion of the fluids which have been carried there. This peristaltic motion throughout the digestive tract is governed by certain muscular fibres, physiologically influenced by the action of Coca, which accounts for its beneficial effect in overcoming constipation.

# Storage Supplies

The average time of the passage of food along the alimentary canal is about twenty-four hours, during which transit it is augmented by several gallons of fluids or juices which are concerned in the process of digestion. There is a constant interchange of these juices from the tissues of the digestive tract and the blood vessels which supply them, absorption taking place wherever there are blood vessels with their accompanying lymphatics, and the tissues of the body are bathed in a sort of lymph at all times even outside of the vessels. Such fluid as may not be directly absorbed into the blood is carried towards the heart and soon becomes part of the circulation, while the refuse is passed off as excreta.

To the liver, which is the largest glandular organ of the body, is attributed a marked influence upon the emotions, an effect really dependent on the fact whether the excreta of the blood are properly converted and eliminated or not. As Henry Ward Beecher said: "When a man's liver is out of order the kingdom of heaven is out of joint," and I presume he knew. Certain it is that there has always been associated with the imperfect action of this organ the idea of despair, which the Greeks presumed due to "black bile" and hence named melancholia /*e\as—black, ^oAx—bile. The liver forms an important function in nutrition not only in the elaboration and purification of the blood, but also in a peculiar property of forming glucose—or a substance akin to sugar or to the starch of plants—which is stored up in the liver cells[14] to be doled out as occasion may demand for the purpose of combustion or the formation of fat.[15] So active is this function that the liver even continues after death to make glycogen, as is termed this first product in its sugar formation.

This animal starch is elaborated chiefly from saccharine or starchy foods, though it is also made from proteids, which are split up into glycogen and urea—a striking example of direct conversion within the body from nitrogenous into a non-nitrogenous substance. The readiness with which the liver forms sugar indicates the possibility of its over production, which is indeed what takes place in glycosuria when the increase of the small amount of sugar which may normally be found in the blood is probably augmented through some nervous impulse and excreted by the kidneys.

The influence of Coca upon nutrition is markedly evidenced by its physiological action, and specifically by the effect of cocaine on glycogen conversion, as demonstrated by the experiments of Ehrlich[16] on the cells of the liver of mice, which under cocaine resembled stuffed goose livers. It should be recalled that the food must be rendered soluble before it can enter the circulation, and once in the blood, if the soluble products of starch—grape sugar, and the soluble peptones from proteids can not be converted into insoluble products they will be swept out of the body through the kidneys. This is precisely what occurs in certain forms of albuminuria and glycosuria. The conversion of similar substances in plant structures under the influence of nitrogenous compounds strongly suggests the utility of the nitrogenous Coca in the conversion of these soluble products into less soluble glycogen and proteids, and indicates a possible application of Coca to the relief of diabetes and albuminuria, disorders in which it has already been employed empirically with advantage.

Man's chief desire is to acquire strength and energy for the furtherance of his ambition, be that of a physical or mental nature. The intelligent being should base his sustenance upon this hopeful instinct. One engaged in active work in the open air usually finds appetite for the food presented without being over fastidious. Throughout the greater part of British India and China the majority of the people live largely upon rice stimulated in its conversion to muscle energy through the nitrogenous influence of a liberal tea drinking. Diametrically opposite on the globe, amidst the cold and rigors of the higher altitude of the Andes the Indian finds his powers effectively sustained by a diet of maize and nitrogenous Coca leaves. Science has verified this crude empirical experience by proving that carbohydrates contribute force when properly converted and that Coca not only creates mental energy, but muscular power through an actual change within the tissue cells. These are facts which it is well to remember.

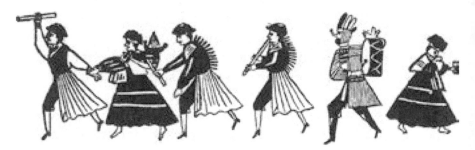

*Bolivian Picture Writing*

Every one realizes that active muscular work provokes fatigue and hunger, but few seem to appreciate that force expenditure is going on within the body all the time. Every movement, be it the most simple, whether the evolution of gentle thought in prayer, the turbulence of passion, even the vital changes incidental to existence, although performed unconsciously, each occasions a conversion of tissue which demands repair. That these functions shall be performed to the end nature has made the brain and nerves imperious in their demand for nourishment. These tissues are chiefly composed of fat and in case of impoverishment every other tissue must yield to their support. First a wasting of the adipose tissue, then the glandular, then the muscles and blood, and if life be further prolonged, brain and nerves would suffer last.

# Influence of Nutrition

Food therefore is essential to maintain bodily repair in mental work as well as in muscular, for brain work indeed is hungry work, even though the pre-occupied worker may forget whether he has dined or not. At such times what might be termed emergency food is desirable to stimulate the flagging forces to activity; a stimulation which we have seen is not done at the expense of essential bodily tissue, for the storage food merely is what is used up, that which has providentially been put away at a period of overproduction to nourish and support in the time of need. It is in this quality that the glycogen in the liver cells or the fat about the muscles acts as a preserver of other tissue.

Fat is not necessarily created from fat, but has its origin in the carbohydrates, and certain fats are desirable according to their digestibility. Pork fat is popularly in bad repute, but the crispy fried bacon, or the fat of boiled ham is really easily digested, while cream, particularly whipped cream, and fresh butter are the most readily assimilated of all edible fats. The chief value of cod liver oil is as a fat food and modern physicians do not prescribe it for patients who can and will take other and more agreeable fats.

Strength and energy are the outgrowths of a proper assimilation in all the functions of the body. There is no one class of food to exclusively nourish any one tissue, but a complex dietary embracing a wide variety is demanded, and is as absolutely necessary for the development of muscle, or brain, or nerve as it is for mere existence itself, for life implies unanimity between all the cells which form the colony of the organism. It is in this sense that Coca is

*Strength and energy are the outgrowths of a proper assimilation in all the functions of the body.* to be regarded as having an important bearing upon nutrition and hence worthy to be ranked among the highest type of stimulants. It is a stimulant to energy, though it does not supply in itself the whole force any more than any other one food can do. In this sense, to borrow an apt simile suggested by Gubler, Coca may be compared to the fulminate of a cartridge, which, though not in itself the force, yet it excites the energy which propels the bullet.[17] As a nitrogenous fulminate is essential to cause the powder to act, so, too, nitrogenous substances are necessary in all metabolism, whether of plant or animal life to provoke nourishment, to stimulate repair and to convert the stored-up substances to activity and usefulness.

There is a foundation of truth when in training a meat diet is adopted—not to make muscle because the meat itself is muscle, but to excite the conversion of stored-up tissue into energy. For this reasom during such a diet flesh is often lost through the using up of stored supplies—but not necessarily of frame work tissue, for the muscles become firmer as the fat is taken from them. It is true that an injudicious dietary may so completely use up this stored tissue that instead of strength there is a lack of power and endurance. This is one example of how mischief may be done by limiting food supplies to one class, which is always an unwise course to follow as a matter of choice for any length of time.

It would seem that the whole idea of "wear and tear" has been popularly misconstrued, and through this misunderstanding there has resulted much mischief. "The body does not waste because it works, but works because it wastes."[18] There is certainly a constant decomposition—a wear and tear—going on in every cell of the tissues, and the more actively these are exercised—within physiological limits— the more rapidly they are renewed. This renewal through activity means life and is absolutely essential to existence.

Food may be stored up, but without its proper conversion there can be no energy and our cells would be simply storehouses of supplies hoarded in a miserly way to no purpose, while death would certainly follow from the encumbrance of surfeit and consequent inertia.

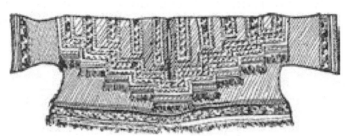

### An Incan Poncho

Unfortunately the body supplies have often been compared to the money saved in a bank, and the excitation to energy through stimulus has been allied to the withdrawal of a certain amount of capital, which, if not immediately returned, must result in impoverishment. This is only theoretical, for if it were literally true the more work the human machine performed the sooner it would be used up, while all know that work—activity—is essential to life and well being, even to rejuvenation and happiness.

If the bodily energies must be compared to a saved-up fund it should be recalled that a bank carries on its affairs by the stimulus of the moneys which pass through it. It does all its work, gives forth an energy of interest, yet holds the capital unimpaired. So the tissues of the human organism are maintained by the stimulus of food, from which there is given forth an interest in energy, while the capital is not necessarily consumed. The mistake, it seems, has arisen from the supposition often advanced that each being is born with a certain life force, just as a steam engine is created capable of a certain amount of work, which may be all consumed in a day or gradually used through a period of years. The modern physiology of cell life emphatically contradicts such a supposition.

The question of the daily amount of food necessarily is a relative one, to be determined by physical development, and the work to be performed. The average amount has been calculated from the daily loss of elements and the proportion of these in the various foodstuffs, a balance being maintained in the relation of the nitrogenous to non-nitrogenous substances, as one to four. It has been estimated that a man weighing one hundred and fifty pounds and in moderate activity will lose somewhere about three hundred grammes of carbon and twenty grammes of nitrogen a day.    Constructing a theoretical diet on this basis the amount of food is selected to approximate this loss. The common error arises in an excess of one or the other of these substances, rather than in too much food, and as satiety gives a sense of satisfaction, the mischief is apt to be overlooked. Every kind of food is capable of maintaining the body for a time and man's high organization admits of ready adaptability, but the necessity for a mixed dietary is founded upon scientific fact. With this thought in view more good may be done by the shaping of an appropriate diet in health than may be accomplished by the most clever wielding of potent remedies in disease.

## Digestive Indiscretions

There is one other factor allied to this matter of dietetics quite as important in regulating assimilation as is the proportion of elements or of comparative digestibility. As all processes and actions are governed by brain power, controlled through nerve conduction, it is essential that the several organs shall not only be fitted, but unimpeded for their functions. In large cities the feverish struggle of daily life more closely concerns money-getting than any elective dietary. This constant nervous tension is a primal cause of digestive disturbance and the long train of evils which follow. Business men as a rule do not take sufficient time to eat, as may be seen in any one of the great restaurants in this city, where the entire feeding of coming and going thousands is sustained in a period almost too brief to admit of enjoying an appropriate meal. The excitement, the hurry and bustle is contagious and the nervous strain reflected is too great to permit of proper digestion. The food is hurried to the stomach improperly prepared, where it must remain as an irritant both to that organ apd the nervous system.

A brain engaged in deep thought cannot properly attend to the digestion of a hearty meal, nor encompassing a hearty meal will the digestive tract permit a brain to give forth its clearest work, both processes must be imperfectly performed when attempted together. The best after dinner speakers commonly only make a pretense of dining when they anticipate that their oratorical efforts are to be called for, while those who, like the Romans, have "dined to the full," fall intothat unargumentative ecstatic condition which dominates a good listener.

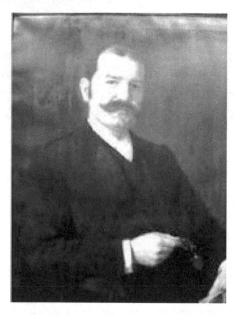

**W. Golden Mortimer** (1854- 1933) received his M.D. from New York University, and a was Fellow of the New York Academy of Medicine, of which his maternal grandfather, James Herring, was a founder. He specialized in diseases of the eye, ear, nose, and throat. As part of his coca studies, Dr. Mortimer became one of the first clinical investigators to systematically query physicians and other professionals in a large-scale inquiry about a drug's effects. The tabulation of the over 1,200 responses he received were published as, "A Collective Investigation Upon the Physiological Action and Therapeutic Application of Coca, Among Several Hundred Physicians."

Before he studied medicine, Dr. Mortimer was a professional magician who toured the U.S. with his show, "Mortimer's Mysteries," from 1869 to 1881. He also worked as a pharmacist in Santa Cruz, California, was the founder and editor of *The Druggist's Advertiser and Trade Journal*, and edited both The Pharmaceutical Journal and The New York Journal of Medicine. Dr. Mortimer also attained the 32nd Degree of Scottish Rite Freemasonry.

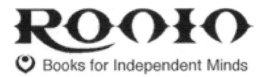
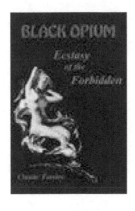
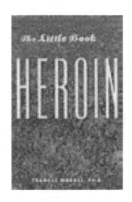
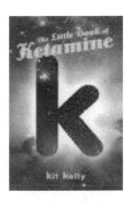
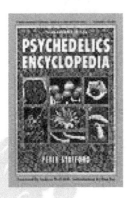
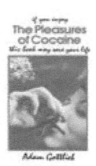
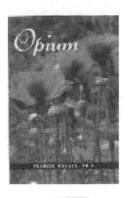

Printed in the USA
CPSIA information can be obtained
at www.ICGtesting.com
JSHW022211140824
68134JS00018B/986